Virtual Clinical Excursions—Medical-Surgical

for

Linton:
Introduction to Medical-Surgical Nursing,
4th Edition

Virtual Clinical Excursions—Medical-Surgical

for

Linton:
Introduction to Medical-Surgical Nursing,
4th Edition

prepared by

Kim D. Cooper, RN, MSN
Ivy Tech Community College
Terre Haute, Indiana

software developed by

Wolfsong Informatics, LLC
Tucson, Arizona

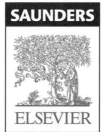
SAUNDERS

ELSEVIER

SAUNDERS
ELSEVIER

11830 Westline Industrial Drive
St. Louis, Missouri 63146

VIRTUAL CLINICAL EXCURSIONS—MEDICAL-SURGICAL FOR
LINTON: INTRODUCTION TO MEDICAL-SURGICAL NURSING
FOURTH EDITION

ISBN: 978-1-4160-4460-4

Copyright © 2007 by Saunders, an imprint of Elsevier Inc.

Notice

Knowledge and best practice in this field are constantly changing. As new research and experience broaden our knowledge, changes in practice, treatment and drug therapy may become necessary or appropriate. Readers are advised to check the most current information provided (i) on procedures featured or (ii) by the manufacturer of each product to be administered, to verify the recommended dose or formula, the method and duration of administration, and contraindications. It is the responsibility of the practitioner, relying on their own experience and knowledge of the patient, to make diagnoses, to determine dosages and the best treatment for each individual patient, and to take all appropriate safety precautions. To the fullest extent of the law, neither the Publisher nor the Authors assumes any liability for any injury and/or damage to persons or property arising out or related to any use of the material contained in this book.

ISBN: 978-1-4160-4460-4

Executive Editor: *Tom Wilhelm*
Managing Editor: *Jeff Downing*
Associate Developmental Editor: *Tiffany Trautwein*
Book Production Manager: *Gayle May*
Project Manager: *Tracey Schriefer*

Printed in the United States of America

Last digit is the print number: 9 8 7 6 5 4 3 2 1

Workbook
prepared by

Kim D. Cooper, RN, MSN
Ivy Tech Community College
Terre Haute, Indiana

Textbook

Adrianne Dill Linton, PhD, RN
Associate Professor
University of Texas Health Science Center at San Antonio
School of Nursing
San Antonio, Texas

Reviewer

Gina Long, RN, DNSc
Assistant Professor, Department of Nursing
College of Health Professions
Northern Arizona University
Flagstaff, Arizona

Contents

Getting Started

Getting Set Up 1

A Quick Tour 9

A Detailed Tour 24

Unit I: Concepts in Nursing Practice

Lesson 1   Cultural Aspects of Nursing Care (Chapter 6) 43

Lesson 2   Nutrition (Chapter 9) 51

Lesson 3   Developmental Processes and the Older Adult (Chapters 10 and 11) 59

Lesson 4   Inflammation, Infection, and Immunity (Chapter 13) 67

Lesson 5   Pain Management (Chapter 15) 75

Lesson 6   Surgical Care (Chapter 17) 85

Lesson 7   Intravenous Therapy (Chapter 18) 95

Lesson 8   Loss, Death, and End-of-Life Care (Chapter 24) 103

Lesson 9   The Patient with Cancer (Chapter 25) 111

Lesson 10   Acute and Chronic Respiratory Disorders (Chapters 30 and 31) 121

Lesson 11   Cardiovascular Disorders: Hypertension (Chapter 37) 137

Lesson 12   Digestive Tract Disorders (Chapter 38) 143

Lesson 13   Connective Tissue Disorders (Chapters 41 and 42) 153

Lesson 14   Endocrine Disorders: Diabetes Mellitus and Hypoglycemia (Chapter 46) 167

Lesson 15   Mental Health and Illness (Chapters 54 and 55) 175

Table of Contents
Linton:
Introduction to Medical-Surgical Nursing, 4th Edition

Unit I: Patient Care Concepts
1   The Health Care System
2   Patient Care Settings
3   Legal and Ethical Considerations
4   The Leadership Role of the Licensed Practical Nurse
5   The Nurse-Patient Relationship
6   Cultural Aspects of Nursing Care
7   The Nurse and the Family
8   Health and Illness
9   Nutrition
10 Developmental Processes
11 The Older Patient
12 The Nursing Process and Critical Thinking

Unit II: Physiologic Responses to Illness
13 Inflammation, Infection, and Immunity
14 Fluid and Electrolytes
15 Pain Management

Unit III: Acute Care
16 First Aid and Emergency Care
17 Surgical Care
18 Intravenous Therapy
19 Shock

Unit IV: Long-Term Care and Home Health Care
20 Falls
21 Immobility
22 Confusion
23 Incontinence
24 Loss, Death, and End-of-Life Care

Unit V: Cancer
25 The Patient with Cancer
26 The Ostomy Patient

Unit VI: Neurologic Disorders
27 Neurologic Disorders
28 Cerebrovascular Accident
29 Spinal Cord Injury

Unit VII: Respiratory Disorders
30 Acute Respiratory Disorders
31 Chronic Respiratory Disorders

Unit VIII: Hematologic and Immunologic Disorders
32   Hematologic Disorders
33   Immunologic Disorders
34   HIV/AIDS

Unit IX: Cardiovascular Disorders
35   Cardiac Disorders
36   Vascular Disorders
37   Hypertension

Unit X: Digestive Disorders
38   Digestive Tract Disorders
39   Disorders of the Liver, Gallbladder, and Pancreas

Unit XI: Urologic Disorders
40   Urologic Disorders

Unit XII: Musculoskeletal Disorders
41   Connective Tissue Disorders
42   Fractures
43   Amputations

Unit XIII: Endocrine Disorders
44   Pituitary and Adrenal Disorders
45   Thyroid and Parathyroid Disorders
46   Diabetes Mellitus and Hypoglycemia

Unit XIV: Reproductive Disorders
47   Female Reproductive Disorders
48   Male Reproductive Disorders
49   Sexually Transmitted Diseases

Unit XV: Integumentary Disorders
50   Skin Disorders

Unit XVI: Disorders of the Eyes, Ears, Nose, and Throat
51   Eye and Vision Disorders
52   Ear and Hearing Disorders
53   Nose Sinus, and Throat Disorders

Unit XVII: Mental Health and Illness
54   Psychological Responses to Illness
55   Psychiatric Disorders
56   Substance-Related Disorders

Appendix A: Abbreviations
Appendix B: ISMP's List of Error-Prone Abbreviations, Symbols, and Dose Designations
Appendix C: Laboratory Reference Values
Appendix D: Spanish-English Health Care Phrases
Appendix E: Answers to Review Questions
Complete Bibliography and Reader References
Glossary

Getting Started

GETTING SET UP

■ **MINIMUM SYSTEM REQUIREMENTS**

WINDOWS™

Windows XP, 2000, 98, ME, NT 4.0 (Recommend Windows XP/2000)
Pentium® III processor (or equivalent) @ 600 MHz (Recommend 800 MHz or better)
128 MB of RAM (Recommend 256 MB or more)
800 x 600 screen size (Recommend 1024 x 768)
Thousands of colors
12x CD-ROM drive
Soundblaster 16 soundcard compatibility
Stereo speakers or headphones

Note: Virtual Clinical Excursions—Medical-Surgical for Windows will require a minimal amount of disk space to install icons and required dll files for Windows 98/ME.

MACINTOSH®

MAC OS X (10.2 or higher)
Apple Power PC G3 @ 500 MHz or better
128 MB of RAM (Recommend 256 MB or more)
800 x 600 screen size (Recommend 1024 x 768)
Thousands of colors
12x CD-ROM drive
Stereo speakers or headphones

1

■ **INSTALLATION INSTRUCTIONS**

WINDOWS™

1. Insert the *Virtual Clinical Excursions—Medical-Surgical* CD-ROM.
2. Inserting the CD should automatically bring up the setup screen if the current product is not already installed.
   a. If the setup screen does not appear automatically (and *Virtual Clinical Excursions—Medical-Surgical* has not been installed already), navigate to the "My Computer" icon on your desktop or in your Start menu.
   b. Double-click on your CD-ROM drive.
   c. If installation does not start at this point:
      (1) Click the **Start** icon on the task bar and select the **Run** option.
      (2) Type d:\setup.exe (where "d:\" is your CD-ROM drive) and press **OK**.
      (3) Follow the onscreen instructions for installation.
3. Follow the onscreen instructions during the setup process.

MACINTOSH®

1. Insert the *Virtual Clinical Excursions—Medical-Surgical* CD in the CD-ROM drive. The disk icon will appear on your desktop.

2. Double-click on the disk icon.

3. Double-click on the MEDICAL-SURGICAL_MAC run file.

Note: Virtual Clinical Excursions—Medical-Surgical for Macintosh does not have an installation setup and can only be run directly from the CD.

■ **HOW TO USE VIRTUAL CLINICAL EXCURSIONS—MEDICAL-SURGICAL**

WINDOWS™

1. Double-click on the *Virtual Clinical Excursions—Medical-Surgical* icon located on your desktop.
2. Or navigate to the program via the Windows Start menu.

Note: Windows 98/ME will require you to restart your computer before running the *Virtual Clinical Excursions—Medical-Surgical* program.

MACINTOSH®

1. Insert the *Virtual Clinical Excursions—Medical-Surgical* CD in the CD-ROM drive. The disk icon will appear on your desktop.

2. Double-click on the disk icon.

3. Double-click on the MEDICAL-SURGICAL_MAC run file.

■ SCREEN SETTINGS

For best results, your computer monitor resolution should be set at a minimum of 800 x 600. The number of colors displayed should be set to "thousands or higher" (High Color or 16 bit) or "millions of colors" (True Color or 24 bit).

Windows™

1. From the **Start** menu, select **Control Panel** (on some systems, you will first go to **Settings**, then to **Control Panel**).
2. Double-click on the **Display** icon.
3. Click on the **Settings** tab.
4. Under **Screen resolution** use the slider bar to select **800 by 600 pixels**.
5. Access the **Colors** drop-down menu by clicking on the down arrow.
6. Select **High Color (16 bit)** or **True Color (24 bit)**.
7. Click on **OK**.
8. You may be asked to verify the setting changes. Click **Yes**.
9. You may be asked to restart your computer to accept the changes. Click **Yes**.

Macintosh®

1. Select the **Monitors** control panel.
2. Select **800 x 600** (or similar) from the **Resolution** area.
3. Select **Thousands** or **Millions** from the **Color Depth** area.

■ WEB BROWSERS

Supported web browsers include Microsoft Internet Explorer (IE) version 6.0 or higher, Netscape version 7.1 or higher, and Mozilla Firefox version 1.4 or higher.

If you use America Online (AOL) for web access, you will need AOL version 4.0 or higher and one of the browsers listed above. Do not use earlier versions of AOL with earlier versions of IE, because you will have difficulty accessing many features.

For best results with AOL:
• Connect to the Internet using AOL version 4.0 or higher.
• Open a private chat within AOL (this allows the AOL client to remain open, without asking whether you wish to disconnect while minimized).
• Minimize AOL.
• Launch a recommended browser.

■ TECHNICAL SUPPORT

Technical support for this product is available between 7:30 a.m. and 7 p.m. (CST), Monday through Friday. Before calling, be sure that your computer meets the minimum system requirements to run this software. Inside the United States and Canada, call 1-800-692-9010. Outside North America, call 314-872-8370. You may also fax your questions to 314-523-4932 or contact Technical Support through e-mail: technical.support@elsevier.com.

ACCESSING *Virtual Clinical Excursions—Medical-Surgical* FROM EVOLVE

The product you have purchased is part of the Evolve family of online courses and learning resources. Please read the following information thoroughly to get started.

To access your instructor's course on Evolve:

Your instructor will provide you with the username and password needed to access this specific course on the Evolve Learning System. Once you have received this information, please follow these instructions:

1. Go to the Evolve student page (http://evolve.elsevier.com/student)

2. Enter your username and password in the **Login to My Evolve** area and click the **Login** button.

3. You will be taken to your personalized **My Evolve** page, where the course will be listed in the **My Courses** module.

TECHNICAL REQUIREMENTS

To use an Evolve course, you will need access to a computer that is connected to the Internet and equipped with web browser software that supports frames. For optimal performance, it is recommended that you have speakers and use a high-speed Internet connection. However, slower dial-up modems (56 K minimum) are acceptable.

Whichever browser you use, the browser preferences must be set to enable cookies and JavaScript and the cache must be set to reload every time.

Enable Cookies

Browser	Steps
Internet Explorer (IE) 6.0 or higher	1. Select **Tools → Internet Options**. 2. Select **Privacy** tab. 3. Use the slider (slide down) to **Accept All Cookies**. 4. Click **OK**. -OR- 3. Click the **Advanced** button. 4. Click the check box next to **Override Automatic Cookie Handling**. 5. Click the **Accept** radio buttons under **First-party Cookies** and **Third-party Cookies**. 6. Click **OK**.
Netscape 7.1 or higher	1. Select **Edit → Preferences**. 2. Select **Privacy & Security**. 3. Select **Cookies**. 4. Select **Enable All Cookies**.
Mozilla Firefox 1.4 or higher	1. Select **Tools → Options**. 2. Select the **Privacy** icon. 3. Click to expand Cookies. 4. Select **Allow sites to set cookies**. 5. Click **OK**.

Enable JavaScript

Browser	Steps
Internet Explorer (IE) 6.0 or higher	1. Select **Tools → Internet Options**. 2. Select **Security** tab. 3. Under **Security level for this zone** set to **Medium** or lower.
Netscape 7.1 or higher	1. Select **Edit → Preferences**. 2. Select **Advanced**. 3. Select **Scripts & Plugins**. 4. Make sure the **Navigator** box is checked to **Enable JavaScript**. 5. Click **OK**.
Mozilla Firefox 1.4 or higher	1. Select **Tools → Options**. 2. Select the **Content** icon. 3. Select **Enable JavaScript**. 4. Click **OK**.

Set Cache to Always Reload a Page

Browser	Steps
Internet Explorer (IE) 6.0 or higher	1. Select **Tools → Internet Options**. 2. Select **General** tab. 3. Go to the **Temporary Internet Files** and click the **Settings** button. 4. Select the radio button for **Every visit to the page** and click **OK** when complete.
Netscape 7.1 or higher	1. Select **Edit → Preferences**. 2. Select **Advanced**. 3. Select **Cache**. 4. Select the **Every time I view the page** radio button. 5. Click **OK**.
Mozilla Firefox 1.4 or higher	1. Select **Tools → Options**. 2. Select the **Privacy** icon. 3. Click to expand Cache. 4. Set the value to "0" in the **Use up to: __ MB of disk space for the cache** field. 5. Click **OK**.

Plug-Ins

 Adobe Acrobat Reader—With the free Acrobat Reader software, you can view and print Adobe PDF files. Many Evolve products offer student and instructor manuals, checklists, and more in this format!

Download at: http://www.adobe.com

 Apple QuickTime—Install this to hear word pronunciations, heart and lung sounds, and many other helpful audio clips within Evolve Online Courses!

Download at: http://www.apple.com

 Adobe Flash Player—This player will enhance your viewing of many Evolve web pages, as well as educational short-form to long-form animation within the Evolve Learning System!

Download at: http://www.adobe.com

 Adobe Shockwave Player—Shockwave is best for viewing the many interactive learning activities within Evolve Online Courses!

Download at: http://www.adobe.com

 Microsoft Word Viewer—With this viewer Microsoft Word users can share documents with those who don't have Word, and users without Word can open and view Word documents. Many Evolve products have testbank, student and instructor manuals, and other documents available for downloading and viewing on your own computer!

Download at: http://www.microsoft.com

 Microsoft PowerPoint Viewer—View PowerPoint 97, 2000, and 2002 presentations even if you don't have PowerPoint with this viewer. Many Evolve products have slides available for downloading and viewing on your own computer!

Download at: http://www.microsoft.com

SUPPORT INFORMATION

Live support is available to customers in the United States and Canada from 7:30 a.m. to 7 p.m. (CST), Monday through Friday by calling **1-800-401-9962**. You can also send an email to evolve-support@elsevier.com.

There is also **24/7 support information** available on the Evolve website (http://evolve.elsevier.com), including:

- Guided Tours
- Tutorials
- Frequently Asked Questions (FAQs)
- Online Copies of Course User Guides
- And much more!

A QUICK TOUR

Welcome to *Virtual Clinical Excursions—Medical-Surgical*, a virtual hospital setting in which you can work with multiple complex patient simulations and also learn to access and evaluate the information resources that are essential for high-quality patient care.

The virtual hospital, Pacific View Regional Hospital, has realistic architecture and access to patient rooms, a Nurses' Station, and a Medication Room.

■ BEFORE YOU START

Make sure you have your textbook nearby when you use the *Virtual Clinical Excursions—Medical-Surgical* CD. You will want to consult topic areas in your textbook frequently while working with the CD and using this workbook.

■ HOW TO SIGN IN

- Enter your name on the Student Nurse identification badge.
- Now choose one of the four periods of care in which to work. In Periods of Care 1 through 3, you can actively engage in patient assessment, entry of data in the electronic patient record (EPR), and medication administration. Period of Care 4 presents the day in review. Highlight and click the appropriate period of care. (For this quick tour, choose **Period of Care 1: 0730-0815**.)
- This takes you to the Patient List screen (see example on page 11). Only the patients on the Medical-Surgical Floor are available. Note that the virtual time is provided in the box at the lower left corner of the screen (0730, since we chose Period of Care 1).

Note: If you choose to work during Period of Care 4: 1900-2000, the Patient List screen is skipped since you are not able to visit patients or administer medications during the shift. Instead, you are taken directly to the Nurses' Station, where the records of all the patients on the floor are available for your review.

■ **PATIENT LIST**

MEDICAL-SURGICAL UNIT

Harry George (Room 401)
Osteomyelitis—A 54-year-old Caucasian male admitted from a homeless shelter with an infected leg. He has complications of type 2 diabetes mellitus, alcohol abuse, nicotine addiction, poor pain control, and complex psychosocial issues.

Jacquline Catanazaro (Room 402)
Asthma—A 45-year-old Caucasian female admitted with an acute asthma exacerbation and suspected pneumonia. She has complications of chronic schizophrenia, noncompliance with medication therapy, obesity, and herniated disc.

Piya Jordan (Room 403)
Bowel obstruction—A 68-year-old Asian female admitted with a colon mass and suspected adenocarcinoma. She undergoes a right hemicolectomy. This patient's complications include atrial fibrillation, hypokalemia, and symptoms of meperidine toxicity.

Clarence Hughes (Room 404)
Degenerative joint disease—A 73-year-old African-American male admitted for a left total knee replacement. His preparations for discharge are complicated by the development of a pulmonary embolus and the need for ongoing intravenous therapy.

Pablo Rodriguez (Room 405)
Metastatic lung carcinoma—A 71-year-old Hispanic male admitted with symptoms of dehydration and malnutrition. He has chronic pain secondary to multiple subcutaneous skin nodules and psychosocial concerns related to family issues with his approaching death.

Patricia Newman (Room 406)
Pneumonia—A 61-year-old Caucasian female admitted with worsening pulmonary function and an acute respiratory infection. Her chronic emphysema is complicated by heavy smoking, hypertension, and malnutrition. She needs access to community resources such as a smoking cessation program and meal assistance.

■ HOW TO SELECT A PATIENT

- You can choose one or more patients to work with from the Patient List by checking the box to the left of the patient name(s). For this quick tour, select Piya Jordan and Pablo Rodriguez. (In order to receive a scorecard for a patient, the patient must be selected before proceeding to the Nurses' Station.)
- Click on **Get Report** to the right of the medical records number (MRN) to view a summary of the patient's care during the 12-hour period before your arrival on the unit.
- After reviewing the report, click on **Return to Patient List** and repeat the previous step to review the report of your second patient.
- When you are ready to begin your care, click on **Go to Nurses' Station** in the right lower corner.

Note: Even though the Patient List is initially skipped when you sign in to work for Period of Care 4, you can still access this screen if you wish to review the shift-change report for any of the patients. To do so, simply click on **Patient List** near the top left corner of the Nurses' Station (or click on the clipboard to the left of the Kardex). Then click on **Get Report** for the patient(s) whose care you are reviewing. This may be done during any period of care.

Patient List

	Patient Name	Room	MRN	Clinical Report
☐	Harry George	401	1868054	Get Report
☐	Jacquline Catanazaro	402	1868048	Get Report
☑	Piya Jordan	403	1868092	Get Report
☐	Clarence Hughes	404	1868011	Get Report
☑	Pablo Rodriguez	405	1868088	Get Report
☐	Patricia Newman	406	1868097	Get Report

Please select all the patients you will be caring for this period of care. Once you have exited the patient list, you will not be able to change your current selections or select new patients to care for.

0730   Go to Nurses' Station

■ HOW TO FIND A PATIENT'S RECORDS

NURSES' STATION

Within the Nurses' Station, you will see:

1. A clipboard that contains the patient list for that floor.
2. A chart rack with patient charts labeled by room number, a notebook labeled Kardex, and a notebook labeled MAR (Medication Administration Record).
3. A desktop computer with access to the Electronic Patient Record (EPR).
4. A tool bar across the top of the screen that can also be used to access the Patient List, EPR, Chart, MAR, and Kardex. This tool bar is also accessible from each patient's room.
5. A Drug Guide containing information about the medications you are able to administer to your patients.
6. A tool bar across the bottom of the screen that you can use to access patient rooms, the Medication Room, the Floor Map, or the Drug Guide.

As you run your cursor over an item, it will be highlighted. To select, simply double-click on the item. As you use these resources, you will always be able to return to the Nurses' Station by clicking on the **Return to Nurses' Station** bar located in the right lower corner of your screen.

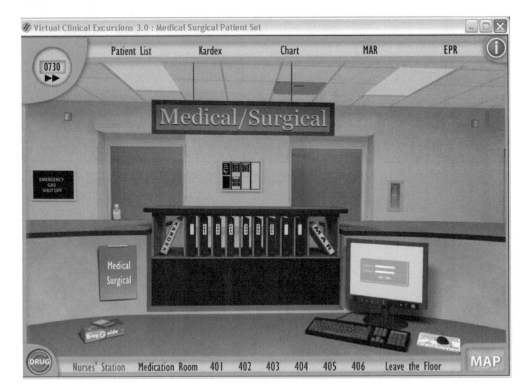

Medication Administration Record (MAR)

The MAR icon located in the tool bar at the top of your screen accesses current 24-hour medications for each patient. Click on the icon and the MAR will open. (*Note:* You can also access the MAR by clicking on the MAR notebook on the far right side of the book rack in the center of the screen.) Within the MAR, tabs on the right side of the screen allow you to select patients by room number. Be careful to make sure you select the correct tab number for *your* patient rather than simply reading the first record that appears after the MAR opens. Each MAR sheet lists the following:

- Medications
- Route and dosage of each medication
- Times of administration of each medication

Note: The MAR changes each day. Expired MARs are stored in the patients' charts.

CHARTS

To access patient charts, either click on the **Chart** icon at the top of your screen or anywhere within the chart rack in the center of the Nurses' Station screen. When the close-up view appears, the individual charts are labeled by room number. To open a chart, click on the room number of the patient whose chart you wish to review. The patient's name and allergies will appear on the left side of the screen, along with a list of tabs on the right side of the screen, allowing you to view the following data:

- Allergies
- Physician's Orders
- Physician's Notes
- Nurse's Notes
- Laboratory Reports
- Diagnostic Reports
- Surgical Reports
- Consultations

- Patient Education
- History and Physical
- Nursing Admission
- Expired MARs
- Consents
- Mental Health
- Admissions
- Emergency Department

Information appears in real time. The entries are in reverse chronologic order, so use the down arrow at the right side of each chart page to scroll down to view previous entries. Flip from tab to tab to view multiple data fields or click on the **Return to Nurses' Station** bar in the lower right corner of the screen to exit the chart.

ELECTRONIC PATIENT RECORD (EPR)

The EPR can be accessed from the computer in the Nurses' Station or from the EPR icon located in the tool bar at the top of your screen. To access a patient's EPR:
- Click on either the computer screen or the **EPR** icon.
- Your username and password are automatically filled in.
- Click on **Login** to enter the EPR.
- *Note:* Like the MAR, the EPR is arranged numerically. Thus when you enter, you are initially shown the records of the patient in the lowest room number on the floor. To view the correct data for *your* patient, remember to select the correct room number, using the drop-down menu for the Patient field at the top left corner of the screen.

The EPR used in Pacific View Regional Hospital represents a composite of commercial versions being used in hospitals. You can access the EPR:
- to review existing data for a patient (by room number).
- to enter data you collect while working with a patient.

The EPR is updated daily, so no matter what day or part of a shift you are working, there will be a current EPR with the patient's data from the past days of the current hospital stay. This type of simulated EPR allows you to examine how data for different attributes have changed over time, as well as to examine data for all of a patient's attributes at a particular time. The EPR is fully functional (as it is in a real-life hospital). You can enter such data as blood pressure, breath sounds, and certain treatments. The EPR will not, however, allow you to enter data for a previous time period. Use the arrows at the bottom of the screen to move forward and backward in time.

Virtual Clinical Excursions 3.0 : Medical Surgical Patient Set				
Patient: 403 **Category:** Vital Signs				**0732**
Name: Piya Jordan	Wed 0630	Wed 0700	Wed 0715	Code Meanings
PAIN: LOCATION		OS		A — Abdomen
PAIN: RATING		5		Ar — Arm
PAIN: CHARACTERISTICS		C		B — Back
PAIN: VOCAL CUES		VC3		C — Chest
PAIN: FACIAL CUES		FC1		Ft — Foot
PAIN: BODILY CUES				H — Head
PAIN: SYSTEM CUES				Hd — Hand
PAIN: FUNCTIONAL EFFECTS				L — Left
PAIN: PREDISPOSING FACTORS				Lg — Leg
PAIN: RELIEVING FACTORS				Lw — Lower
PCA		P		N — Neck
TEMPERATURE (F)		99.6		NN — See Nurses notes
TEMPERATURE (C)				OS — Operative site
MODE OF MEASUREMENT		Ty		Or — See Physicians orders
SYSTOLIC PRESSURE		110		PN — See Progress notes
DIASTOLIC PRESSURE		70		R — Right
BP MODE OF MEASUREMENT		NIBP		Up — Upper
HEART RATE		104		
RESPIRATORY RATE		18		
SpO2 (%)		95		
BLOOD GLUCOSE				
WEIGHT				
HEIGHT				

◀   ▶   Exit EPR

At the top of the EPR screen, you can choose patients by their room numbers. In addition, you have access to 17 different categories of patient data. To change patients or data categories, click the down arrow to the right of the room number or category.

The categories of patient data in the EPR as as follows:

- Vital Signs
- Respiratory
- Cardiovascular
- Neurologic
- Gastrointestinal
- Excretory
- Musculoskeletal
- Integumentary
- Reproductive
- Psychosocial
- Wounds and Drains
- Activity
- Hygiene and Comfort
- Safety
- Nutrition
- IV
- Intake and Output

Remember, each hospital selects its own codes. The codes used in the EPR at Pacific View Regional Hospital may be different from ones you have seen in your clinical rotations. Take some time to acquaint yourself with the codes. Within the Vital Signs category, click on any item in the left column (e.g., Pain: Characteristics). In the far-right column, you will see a list of code meanings for the possible findings and/or descriptors for that assessment area.

You will use the codes to record the data you collect as you work with patients. Click on the box in the last time column to the right of any item and wait for the code meanings applicable to that entry to appear. Select the appropriate code to describe your assessment findings and type it in the box. (*Note:* If no cursor appears within the box, click on the box again until the blue shading disappears and the blinking cursor appears.) Once the data are typed in this box, they are entered into the patient's record for this period of care only.

To leave the EPR, click on **Exit EPR** in the bottom right corner of the screen.

■ VISITING A PATIENT

From the Nurses' Station, click on the room number of the patient you wish to visit in the tool bar at the bottom of your screen. Once you are inside the room, you will see a still photo of your patient in the top left corner. To verify that this is the patient you have chosen, click on the **Check Armband** icon to the right of the photo. The patient's identification data will appear. If you click on **Check Allergies** (the next icon to the right), a list of the patient's allergies (if any) will replace the photo.

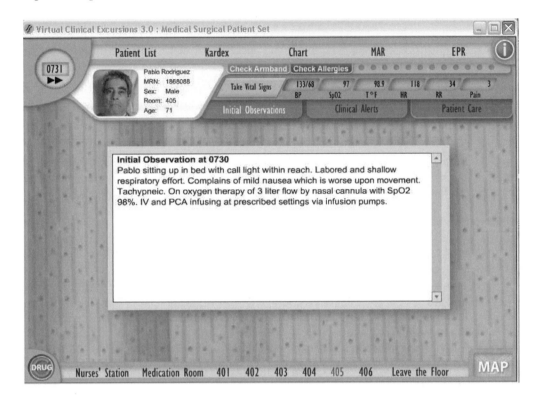

Also located in the patient's room are multiple icons you can use to assess the patient or the patient's medications. A virtual clock is provided in the upper left corner of the room to monitor your progress in real time. (*Note:* The fast-forward icon within the virtual clock will advance the time by 2-minute intervals when clicked.)

- The tool bar across the top of the screen allows you to check the **Patient List**, access the **EPR** to check or enter data, and view the patient's **Chart**, **MAR**, or **Kardex**.

- The **Take Vital Signs** icon allows you to measure the patient's up-to-the-minute blood pressure, oxygen saturation, temperature, heart rate, respiratory rate, and pain level.

- Each time you enter a patient's room, you are given an Initial Observation report to review (in the text box under the patient's photo). These notes are provided to give you a "look" at the patient as if you had just stepped into the room. You can also click on the **Initial Observations** icon to return to this box from other views within the patient's room. To the right of this icon is **Clinical Alerts**, a resource that allows you to make decisions about priority medication interventions based on emerging data collected in real time. Check this screen throughout your period of care to avoid missing critical information related to recently ordered or STAT medications.

- Clicking on the **Patient Care** icon opens up three specific learning environments within the patient room: **Physical Assessment**, **Nurse-Client Interactions**, and **Medication Administration**.

- To perform a **Physical Assessment**, choose a body area (such as **Head & Neck**) by clicking on the appropriate icon in the column of yellow buttons. This activates a list of system sub-categories for that body area (e.g., see **Sensory**, **Neurologic**, etc. in the green boxes). After you click on the system that you wish to evaluate, a still photo and text box appear, describing the assessment findings. The still photo is a "snapshot" of how an assessment of this area might be done or what the finding might look like. For every body area, there is also an **Equipment** button located on the far right of the screen.

- To the right of the Physical Assessment icon is **Nurse-Client Interactions**. Clicking on this icon will reveal the times and titles of any videos available for viewing. (*Note:* If the video you wish to see is not listed, this means you have not yet reached the correct virtual time to view that video. Check the virtual clock; you may return to access the video once its designated time has occurred—as long as you do so within the same period of care. Or you can click on the fast-forward icon within the virtual clock to advance the time by 2-minute intervals. You will then need to click again on **Patient Care** and **Nurse-Client Interactions** to refresh the screen.) To view a listed video, click on the white arrow to the right of the video title. Use the control buttons below the video to start, stop, pause, rewind, or fast-forward the action or to mute the sound.

- **Medication Administration** is the pathway that allows you to review and administer medications to a patient after you have prepared them in the Medication Room. This process is addressed further in the *How to Prepare Medications* section (pages 19-20) and in *Medications* (pages 26-30). For additional hands-on practice, see *Reducing Medication Errors* (pages 37-41).

■ **HOW TO QUIT, CHANGE PATIENTS, OR CHANGE PERIOD OF CARE**

How to Quit: From most screens, you may click the **Leave the Floor** icon on the bottom tool bar to the right of the patient room numbers. (*Note:* From some screens, you will first need to click an **Exit** button or **Return to Nurses' Station** before clicking **Leave the Floor**.) When the Floor Menu appears, click **Exit** to leave the program.

How to Change Patients or Period of Care: To change patients, simply click on the new patient's room number. (You cannot receive a scorecard for a new patient, however, unless you have already selected that patient on the Patient List screen.) To change to a new period of care or to restart the virtual clock, click on **Leave the Floor** and then on **Restart the Program**.

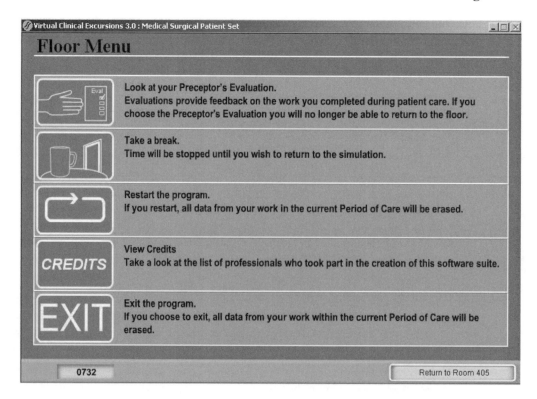

■ HOW TO PREPARE MEDICATIONS

From the Nurses' Station or the patient's room, you can access the Medication Room by clicking on the icon in the tool bar at the bottom of your screen to the left of the patient room numbers.

In the Medication Room you have access to the following (from left to right):

- A preparation area is located on the counter under the cabinets. To begin the medication preparation process, click on the tray on the counter or click on the **Preparation** icon at the top of the screen. The next screen leads you through a specific sequence (called the Preparation Wizard) to prepare medications one at a time for administration to a patient. However, no medication has been selected at this time. We will do this while working with a patient in *A Detailed Tour*. To exit this screen, click on **View Medication Room**.

- To the right of the cabinets (and above the refrigerator), IV storage bins are provided. Click on the bins themselves or on the **IV Storage** icon at the top of the screen. The bins are labeled **Microinfusion**, **Small Volume**, and **Large Volume**. Click on an individual bin to see a list of its contents. If you needed to prepare an IV medication at this time, you could click on the medication and its label would appear to the right under the patient's name. Next, you would click **Put Medication on Tray**. If you ever change your mind or choose the incorrect medication, you can reverse your actions by clicking on **Put Medication in Bin**. Click **Close Bin** in the right bottom corner to exit. **View Medication Room** brings you back to a full view of the entire room.

- A refrigerator is located under the IV storage bins to hold any medications that must be stored below room temperature. Click on the refrigerator door or on the **Refrigerator** icon at the top of the screen. Then click on the close-up view of the door to access the medications. When you are finished, click **Close Door** and then **View Medication Room**.

- To prepare controlled substances, click the **Automated System** icon at the top of the screen or click the computer monitor located to the right of the IV storage bins. A login screen will appear; your name and password are automatically filled in. Click **Login**. Select the patient for whom you wish to access medications; then select the correct medication drawer to open (they are stored alphabetically). Click **Open Drawer**, highlight the proper medication, and choose **Put Medication on Tray**. When you are finished, click **Close Drawer** and then **View Medication Room**.

- Next to the Automated System is a set of drawers identified by patient room number. To access these, click on the drawers themselves or on the **Unit Dosage** icon at the top of the screen. This provides a close-up view of the drawers. To open a drawer, click on the room number of the patient you are working with. Next, click on the medication you would like to prepare for the patient, and a label will appear to the right, listing the medication strength, units, and dosage per unit. You can **Open** and **Close** this medication label by clicking the appropriate icon. To exit, click **Close Drawer**; then click **View Medication Room**.

At any time, you can learn about a medication you wish to prepare for a patient by clicking on the **Drug** icon in the bottom left corner of the medication room screen or by clicking the **Drug Guide** book on the counter to the right of the unit dosage drawers. The **Drug Guide** provides information about the medications commonly included in nursing drug handbooks. Nutritional supplements and maintenance intravenous fluid preparations are not included.

To access the MAR to review the medications ordered for a patient, click on the **MAR** icon located in the tool bar at the top of your screen and then click on the correct tab for your patient's room number. You may also click the **Review MAR** icon in the tool bar at the bottom of your screen from inside each medication storage area.

After you have chosen and prepared your medications, return to the patient's room to administer them by clicking on the room number in the bottom tool bar. Once inside the patient's room, click on **Patient Care** and then on **Medication Administration** and follow the proper administration sequence.

■ PRECEPTOR'S EVALUATIONS

When you have finished a session, click on **Leave the Floor** to go to the Floor Menu. At this point, you can click on the top icon (**Look at Your Preceptor's Evaluation**) to receive a score-card that provides feedback on the work you completed during patient care.

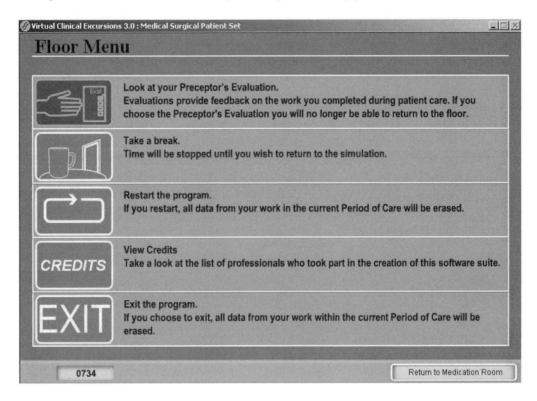

Evaluations are available for each patient you selected when you signed in for the current period of care. Click on the **Medication Scorecard** icon to see an example.

The scorecard compares the medications you administered to a patient during a period of care with what should have been administered. Table A lists the correct medications. Table B lists any medications that were administered incorrectly.

Remember, not every medication listed on the MAR should necessarily be given. For example, a patient might have an allergy to a drug that was ordered, or a medication might have been improperly transcribed to the MAR. Predetermined medication "errors" embedded within the program challenge you to exercise critical thinking skills and professional judgment when deciding to administer a medication, just as you would in a real hospital. Use all your available resources, such as the patient's chart and the MAR, to make your decision.

Table C lists the resources that were available to assist you in medication administration. It also documents whether and when you accessed these resources. For example, did you check the patient armband or perform a check of vital signs? If so, when?

You can click **Print** to get a copy of this report if needed. When you have finished reviewing the scorecard, click **Return to Evaluations** and then **Return to Menu**.

■ **FLOOR MAP**

To get a general sense of your location within the hospital, you can click on the **Map** icon found in the lower right corner of most of the screens in the *Virtual Clinical Excursions—Medical-Surgical* program. (*Note:* If you are following this quick tour step by step, you will need to **Restart the Program** from the Floor Menu, sign in again, and go to the Nurses' Station to access the map.) When you click the **Map** icon, a floor map appears, showing the layout of the floor you are currently on, as well as a directory of the patients and services on that floor. As you move your cursor over the directory list, the location of each room is highlighted on the map (and vice versa). The floor map can be accessed from the Nurses' Station, Medication Room, and each patient's room.

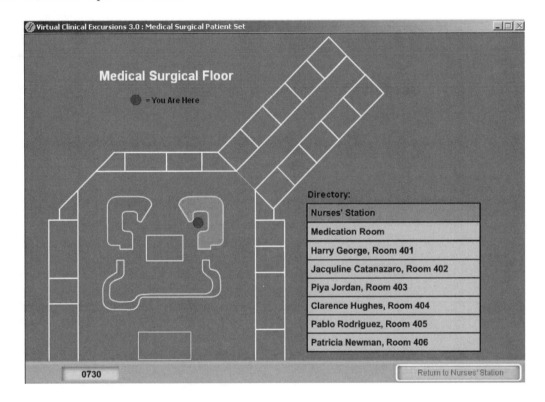

A DETAILED TOUR

If you wish to more thoroughly understand the capabilities of *Virtual Clinical Excursions—Medical-Surgical*, take a detailed tour by completing the following section. During this tour, we will work with a specific patient to introduce you to all the different components and learning opportunities available within the software.

■ WORKING WITH A PATIENT

Sign in for Period of Care 1 (0730-0815). From the Patient List, select Piya Jordan in Room 403; however, do not go to the Nurses' Station yet.

■ REPORT

In hospitals, when one shift ends and another begins, the outgoing nurse who attended a patient will give a verbal and sometimes a written summary of that patient's condition to the incoming nurse who will assume care for the patient. This summary is called a report and is an important source of data to provide an overview of a patient. Your first task is to get the clinical report on Piya Jordan. To do this, click **Get Report** in the far right column in this patient's row. From a brief review of this summary, identify the problems and areas of concern that you will need to address for this patient.

When you have finished noting any areas of concern, click **Go to Nurses' Station**.

■ CHARTS

You can access Piya Jordan's chart from the Nurses' Station or from the patient's room (403). We will access it from the Nurses' Station: Click on the chart rack or on the **Chart** icon in the tool bar at the top of your screen. Next, click on the chart labeled **403** to open the medical record for Piya Jordan. Click on the **Emergency Department** tab to view a record of why this patient was admitted.

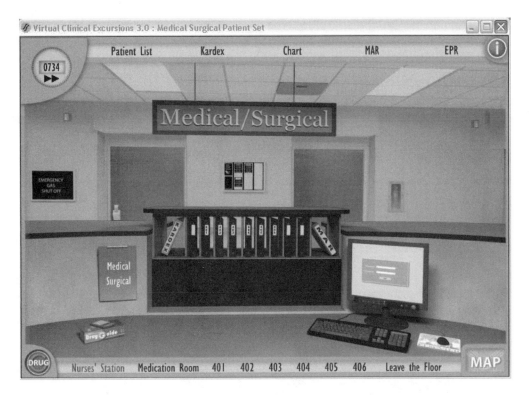

How many days has Piya Jordan been in the hospital?

What tests were done upon her arrival in the Emergency Department and why?

What was her reason for admission?

You should also click on **Surgical Reports** to learn what procedures were performed and when. Finally, review the **Nursing Admission** and **History and Physical** to learn about the health history of this patient. When you are done reviewing the chart, click **Return to Nurses' Station**.

■ MEDICATIONS

Open the Medication Administration Record (MAR) by clicking on the **MAR** icon in the tool bar at the top of your screen. *Remember:* The MAR automatically opens to the first occupied room number on the floor—which is not necessarily your patient's room number! Since you need to access Piya Jordan's MAR, click on tab **403** (her room number). Always make sure you are giving the *Right Drug to the Right Patient!*

Examine the list of medications ordered for Piya Jordan. In the table below, list the medications that need to be given during this period of care (0730-0815). For each medication, note the dosage, route, and time to be given.

Time	Medication	Dosage	Route

Click on **Return to Nurses' Station**. Next, click on **403** on the bottom tool bar and then verify that you are indeed in Piya Jordan's room. Select **Clinical Alerts** (the icon to the right of Initial Observations) to check for any emerging data that might affect your medication administration priorities. Next, go to the patient's chart (click on the **Chart** icon; then click on **403**). When the chart opens, select the **Physician's Orders** tab.

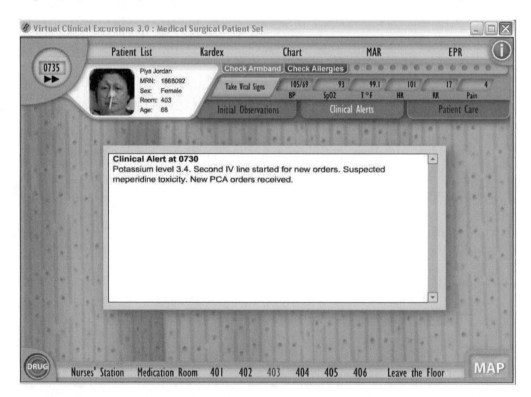

Review the orders. Have any new medications been ordered? Return to the MAR (click **Return to Room 403**; then click **MAR**). Verify that the new medications have been correctly transcribed to the MAR. Mistakes are sometimes made in the transcription process in the hospital setting, and it is sound practice to double-check any new order.

Are there any patient assessments you will need to perform before administering these medications? If so, return to Room 403 and click on **Patient Care** and then **Physical Assessment** to complete those assessments before proceeding.

Now click on the **Medication Room** icon in the tool bar at the bottom of your screen to locate and prepare the medications for Piya Jordan.

In the Medication Room, you must access the medications for Piya Jordan from the specific dispensing system in which each medication is stored. Locate each medication that needs to be given in this time period and click on **Put Medication on Tray** as appropriate. (*Hint:* Look in Unit Dosage drawer first.) When you are finished, click on **Close Drawer** and then on **View Medication Room**. Now click on the medication tray on the counter on the left side of the medication room screen to begin preparing the medications you have selected. (*Remember:* You can also click **Preparation** in the tool bar at the top of the screen.)

In the preparation area, you should see a list of the medications you put on the tray in the previous steps. Click on the first medication and then click **Prepare**. Follow the onscreen instructions of the Preparation Wizard, providing any data requested. As an example, let's follow the preparation process for digoxin, one of the medications due to be administered to Piya Jordan during this period of care. To begin, click to select **Digoxin**; then click **Prepare**. Now work through the Preparation Wizard sequence as detailed below:

> Amount of medication in the ampule: 2 mL.
> Enter the amount of medication you will draw up into a syringe: **0.5** mL.
> Click **Next**.
> Select the patient you wish to set aside the medication for: **Room 403, Piya Jordan**.
> Click **Finish**.
> Click **Return to Medication Room**.

Follow this same basic process for the other medications due to be administered to Piya Jordan during this period of care. (*Hint:* Look in **IV Storage** and **Automated System**.)

PREPARATION WIZARD EXCEPTIONS

- Some medications in *Virtual Clinical Excursions—Medical-Surgical* are preprepared by the pharmacy (e.g., IV antibiotics) and taken to the patient room as a whole. This is common practice in most hospitals.
- Blood products are not administered by students through the *Virtual Clinical Excursions—Medical-Surgical* simulations since blood administration follows specific protocols not covered in this program.
- The *Virtual Clinical Excursions—Medical-Surgical* simulations do not allow for mixing more than one type of medication, such as regular and Lente insulins, in the same syringe. In the clinical setting, when multiple types of insulin are ordered for a patient, the regular insulin is drawn up first, followed by the longer-acting insulin. Insulin is always administered in a special unit-marked syringe.

Now return to Room 403 (click on **403** on the bottom tool bar) to administer Piya Jordan's medications.

At any time during the medication administration process, you can perform a further review of systems, take vital signs, check information contained within the chart, or verify patient identity and allergies. Inside Piya Jordan's room, click **Take Vital Signs**. (*Note:* These findings change over time to reflect the temporal changes you would find in a patient similar to Piya Jordan.)

When you have gathered all the data you need, click on **Patient Care** and then select **Medication Administration**. Any medications you prepared in the previous steps should be listed on the left side of your screen. Let's continue the administration process with the digoxin ordered for Piya Jordan. Click to highlight **Digoxin** in the list of medications. Next, click on the down arrow to the right of **Select** and choose **Administer** from the drop-down menu. This will activate the Administration Wizard. Complete the Wizard sequence as follows:

- Route: **IV**
- Method: **Direct Injection**
- Site: **Peripheral IV**
- Click **Administer to Patient** arrow.
- Would you like to document this administration in the MAR? **Yes**
- Click **Finish** arrow.

Your selections are recorded by a tracking system and evaluated on a Medication Scorecard stored under Preceptor's Evaluations. This scorecard can be viewed, printed, and given to your instructor. To access the Preceptor's Evaluations, click on **Leave the Floor**. When the Floor Menu appears, click on the icon next to **Look at Your Preceptor's Evaluation**. Then click on **Medication Scorecard** inside the box with Piya Jordan's name (see example on the following page).

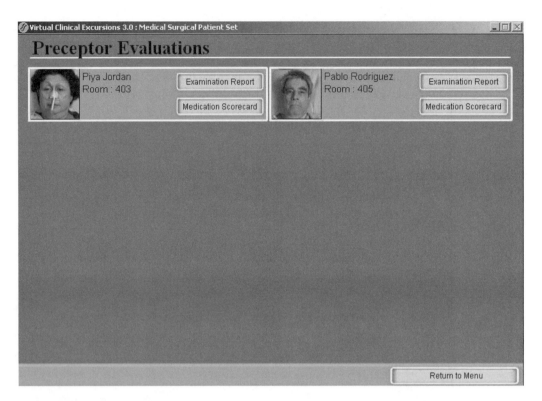

■ MEDICATION SCORECARD

- First, review Table A. Was digoxin given correctly? Did you give the other medications as ordered?
- Table B shows you which (if any) medications you gave incorrectly.
- Table C addresses the resources used for Piya Jordan. Did you access the patient's chart, MAR, EPR, or Kardex as needed to make safe medication administration decisions?
- Did you check the patient's armband to verify her identity? Did you check whether your patient had any known allergies to medications? Were vital signs taken?

When you have finished reviewing the scorecard, click **Return to Evaluations** and then **Return to Menu**.

■ VITAL SIGNS

Vital signs, often considered the traditional "signs of life," include body temperature, heart rate, respiratory rate, blood pressure, oxygen saturation of the blood, and pain level.

Inside Piya Jordan's room, click **Take Vital Signs**. (*Note:* If you are following this detailed tour step by step, you will need to **Restart the Program** from the Floor Menu, sign in again, and navigate to Room 403.) Collect vital signs for this patient and record them in the following table. Note the time at which you collected each of these data. (*Remember:* You can take vital signs at any time. The data change over time to reflect the temporal changes you would find in a patient similar to Piya Jordan.)

Vital Signs	Findings/Time
Blood pressure	
O$_2$ saturation	
Heart rate	
Respiratory rate	
Temperature	
Pain rating	

After you are done, click on the **EPR** icon located in the tool bar at the top of the screen. Your username and password are automatically provided. Click on **Login** to enter the EPR. To access Piya Jordan's records, click on the down arrow next to Patient and choose her room number, **403**. Select **Vital Signs** as the category. Next, in the empty time column on the far right, record the vital signs data you just collected in Piya Jordan's room. (*Note:* If you need help with this process, see page 16.) Now compare these findings with the data you collected earlier for this patient's vital signs. Use these earlier findings to establish a baseline for each of the vital signs.

    a.   Are any of the data you collected significantly different from the baseline for a particular vital sign?

        Circle One: Yes   No

    b.   If "Yes," which data are different?

■ PHYSICAL ASSESSMENT

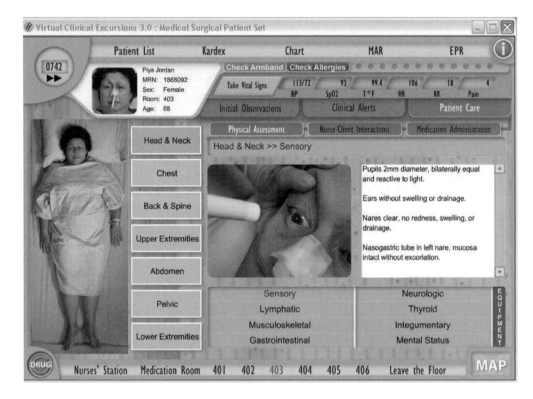

After you have finished examining the EPR for vital signs, click **Exit EPR** to return to Room 403. Click **Patient Care** and then **Physical Assessment**. Think about what information you received in the report at the beginning of this shift, as well as what you may have learned about this patient from the chart. Based on this, what area(s) of examination should you pay most attention to at this time? Is there any equipment you should be monitoring? Conduct a physical assessment of the body areas and systems that you consider priorities for Piya Jordan. For example, select **Head & Neck**; then click on and assess **Sensory** and **Lymphatic**. Complete any other assessment(s) you think are necessary at this time. In the following table, record the data you collected during this examination.

Area of Examination	Findings
Head & Neck Sensory	
Head & Neck Lymphatic	

After you have finished collecting these data, return to the EPR. Compare the data that were already in the record with those you just collected.

a. Are any of the data you collected significantly different from the baselines for this patient?

Circle One: Yes   No

b. If "Yes," which data are different?

■ **NURSE-CLIENT INTERACTIONS**

Click on **Patient Care** from inside Piya Jordan's room (403). Now click on **Nurse-Client Interactions** to access a short video titled **Pain—Adverse Drug Event**, which is available for viewing at or after 0735 (based on the virtual clock in the upper left corner of your screen; see *Note* below). To begin the video, click on the arrow next to its title. You will observe a nurse communicating with Piya Jordan and her daughter. There are many variations of nursing practice, some exemplifying "best" practice and some not. Note whether the nurse in this interaction displays professional behavior and compassionate care. Are her words congruent with what is going on with the patient? Does this interaction "feel right" to you? If not, how would you handle this situation differently? Explain.

Note: If the video you wish to view is not listed, this means you have not yet reached the correct virtual time to view that video. Check the virtual clock; you may return to access the video once its designated time has occurred—as long as you do so within the same period of care. Or you can click on the fast-forward icon within the virtual clock to advance the time by 2-minute intervals. You will then need to click again on **Patient Care** and **Nurse-Client Interactions** to refresh the screen.

At least one Nurse-Client Interactions video is available during each period of care. Viewing these videos can help you learn more about what is occurring with a patient at a certain time and also prompt you to discern between nurse communications that are ideal and those that need improvement. Compassionate care and the ability to communicate clearly are essential components of delivering quality nursing care, and it is during your clinical time that you will begin to refine these skills.

■ COLLECTING AND EVALUATING DATA

Each of the activities you perform in the Patient Care environment generates a significant amount of assessment data. Remember that after you collect data, you can record your findings in the EPR. You can also review the EPR, patient's chart, videos, and MAR at any time. You will get plenty of practice collecting and then evaluating data in context of the patient's course.

Now, here's an important question for you:

> Did the previous sequence of exercises provide the most efficient way to assess
> Piya Jordan?

For example, you went to the patient's room to get vital signs, then back to the EPR to enter data and compare your findings with extant data. Next, you went back to the patient's room to do a physical examination, then again back to the EPR to enter and review data. If this back-and-forth process of data collection and recording seemed inefficient, remember the following:

- Plan all of your nursing activities to maximize efficiency, while at the same time optimizing the quality of patient care. (Think about what data you might need before performing certain tasks. For example, do you need to check a heart rate before administering a cardiac medication or check an IV site before starting an infusion?)

- You collect a tremendous amount of data when you work with a patient. Very few people can accurately remember all these data for more than a few minutes. Develop efficient assessment skills, and record data as soon as possible after collecting them.

- Assessment data are only the starting point for the nursing process.

Make a clear distinction between these first exercises and how you actually provide nursing care. These initial exercises were designed to involve you actively in the use of different software components. This workbook focuses on sensible practices for implementing the nursing process in ways that ensure the highest-quality care of patients.

Most important, remember that a human being changes through time, and that these changes include both the physical and psychosocial facets of a person as a living organism. Think about this for a moment. Some patients may change physically in a very short time (a patient with emerging myocardial infarction) or more slowly (a patient with a chronic illness). Patients' overall physical and psychosocial conditions may improve or deteriorate. They may have effective coping skills and familial support, or they may feel alone and full of despair. In fact, each individual is a complex mix of physical and psychosocial elements, and at least some of these elements usually change through time.

Thus it is crucial that you *DO NOT* think of the nursing process as a simple one-time, five-step procedure consisting of assessment, nursing diagnosis, planning, implementation, and evaluation. Rather, the nursing process should be utilized as a creative and systematic approach to delivering nursing care. Furthermore, because all living organisms are constantly changing, we must apply the nursing process over and over. Each time we follow the nursing process for an individual patient, we refine our understanding of that patient's physical and psychosocial conditions based on collection and analysis of many different types of data. *Virtual Clinical Excursions—Medical-Surgical* will help you develop both the creativity and the systematic approach needed to become a nurse who is equipped to deliver the highest-quality care to all patients.

REDUCING MEDICATION ERRORS ―――――――――――――――

Earlier in this detailed tour, you learned the basic steps of medication preparation and administration. The following simulations will allow you to practice those skills further—with an increased emphasis on reducing medication errors by using the Medication Scorecard to evaluate your work.

Sign in to work at Pacific View Regional Hospital for Period of Care 1. (*Note:* If you are already working with another patient or during another period of care, click on **Leave the Floor** and then **Restart the Program**; then sign in.)

From the Patient List, select Clarence Hughes. Then click on **Go to Nurses' Station**. Complete the following steps to prepare and administer medications to Clarence Hughes.

- Click on **Medication Room**.
- Click on **MAR** and then on tab **404** to determine prn medications that have been ordered for Clarence Hughes to address his constipation and pain. (*Note:* You may click on **Review MAR** at any time to verify the correct medication order. Always remember to check the patient name on the MAR to make sure you have the correct patient's record—you must click on the correct room number tab within the MAR.) Click on **Return to Medication Room** after reviewing the correct MAR.
- Click on **Unit Dosage** (or on the Unit Dosage cabinet); from the close-up view, click on drawer **404**.
- Select the medications you would like to administer. After each selection, click **Put Medication on Tray**. When you are finished selecting medications, click **Close Drawer** and then **View Medication Room**.
- Click on **Automated System** (or on the Automated System unit itself). Click **Login**.
- On the next screen, specify the correct patient and drawer location.
- Select the medication you would like to administer and click on **Put Medication on Tray**. Repeat this process if you wish to administer other medications from the Automated System.
- When you are finished, click **Close Drawer** and **View Medication Room**.
- From the Medication Room, click on **Preparation** (or on the preparation tray).
- From the list of medications on your tray, highlight the correct medication to administer and click **Prepare**.
- This activates the Preparation Wizard. Supply any requested information; then click **Next**.
- Now select the correct patient to receive this medication and click **Finish**.
- Repeat the previous three steps until all medications that you want to administer are prepared.
- You can click on **Review Your Medications** and then on **Return to Medication Room** when ready. Once you are back in the Medication Room, go directly to Clarence Hughes' room by clicking on **404** at bottom of screen.
- Inside the patient's room, administer the medication, utilizing the five rights of medication administration. After you have collected the appropriate assessment data and are ready for administration, click **Patient Care** and then **Medication Administration**. Verify that the correct patient and medication(s) appear in the left-hand window. Highlight the first medication you wish to administer; then click the down arrow next to Select. From the drop-down menu, select **Administer** and complete the Administration Wizard by providing any information requested. When the Wizard stops asking for information, click **Administer to Patient**. Specify **Yes** when asked whether this administration should be recorded in the MAR. Finally, click **Finish**.

■ SELF-EVALUATION

Now let's see how you did during your medication administration!

- Click on **Leave the Floor** at the bottom of your screen. From the Floor Menu, select **Look at Your Preceptor's Evaluation**. Then click on **Medication Scorecard** for Clarence Hughes. These resources will help you find out more about each patient's medications and possible sources of medication errors.

1. Start by examining Table A. These are the medications you should have given to Clarence Hughes during this period of care. If each of the medications in Table A has a √ by it, then you made no errors. Congratulations!

If any medication has an X by it, then you made one or more medication errors.

Compare Tables A and B to determine which of the following types of errors you made: Wrong Dose, Wrong Route/Method/Site, or Wrong Time. Follow these steps:
   a. Find medications in Table A that were given incorrectly.
   b. Now see if those same medications are in Table B, which shows what you actually administered to Clarence Hughes.
   c. Comparing Tables A and B, match the Strength, Dose, Route/Method/Site, and Time for each medication you administered incorrectly.
   d. Then, using the form below, list the medications given incorrectly and mark the errors you made for each medication.

Medication	Strength	Dosage	Route	Method	Site	Time
	❑	❑	❑	❑	❑	❑
	❑	❑	❑	❑	❑	❑
	❑	❑	❑	❑	❑	❑
	❑	❑	❑	❑	❑	❑

2. To help you reduce future medication errors, consider the following list of possible reasons for errors.

- Did not check drug against MAR for correct patient, correct date, correct time, correct drug, and correct dose.
- Did not check drug dose against MAR three times.
- Did not open the unit dose package in the patient's room.
- Did not correctly identify the patient using two identifiers.
- Did not administer the drug on time.
- Did not verify patient allergies.
- Did not check the patient's current condition or vital sign parameters.
- Did not consider why the patient would be receiving this drug.
- Did not question why the drug was in the patient's drawer.
- Did not check the physician's order and/or check with the pharmacist when there was a question about the drug or dose.
- Did not verify that no adverse effects had occurred from a previous dose.

Based on these possibilities, determine how you made each error and record the reason into the form below:

Medication	Reason for Error

3. Look again at Table B. Are there medications listed that are not in Table A? If so, you gave a medication to Clarence Hughes that he should not have received. Complete the following exercises to help you understand how such an error might have been made.

a. Perhaps you gave a medication that was on Clarence Hughes' MAR for this period of care, without recognizing that a change had occurred in the patient's condition, which should have caused you to reconsider. Review patient records as necessary and complete the following form:

Medication	Possible Reasons Not to Give This Medication

b. Another possibility is that you gave Clarence Hughes a medication that should have been given at a different time. Check his MAR and complete the form below to determine whether you made a Wrong Time error:

Medication	Given to Clarence Hughes at What Time	Should Have Been Given at What Time

c. Maybe you gave another patient's medication to Clarence Hughes. In this case, you made a Wrong Patient error. Check the MARs of other patients and use the form below to determine whether you made this type of error:

Medication	Given to Clarence Hughes	Should Have Been Given to

4. The Medication Scorecard provides some other interesting sources of information. For example, if there is a medication selected for Clarence Hughes but it was not given to him, there will be an X by that medication in Table A, but it will not appear in Table B. In that case, you might have given this medication to some other patient, which is another type of Wrong Patient error. To investigate further, look at Table D, which lists the medications you gave to other patients. See whether you can find any medications for Clarence Hughes that were given to another patient by mistake. However, before you make any decisions, be sure to cross-check the MAR for other patients because the same medication may have been ordered for multiple patients. Use the following form to record your findings:

Medication	Should Have Been Given to Clarence Hughes	Given by Mistake to

5. Now take some time to review the medication exercises you just completed. Use the form below to create an overall analysis of what you have learned. Once again, record each of the medication errors you made, including the type of each error. Then, for each error you made, indicate specifically what you would do differently to prevent this type of error from occurring again.

Medication	Type of Error	Error Prevention Tactic

Submit this form to your instructor if required as a graded assignment, or simply use these exercises to improve your understanding of medication errors and how to reduce them.

Name: _____   Date: _____

The following icons are used throughout the workbook to help you quickly identify particular activities and assignments:

 Indicates a reading assignment—tells you which textbook chapter(s) you should read before starting each lesson

 Indicates a writing activity

 Marks the beginning of an interactive CD-ROM activity—signals you to open or return to your *Virtual Clinical Excursions—Medical-Surgical* CD-ROM

 Indicates additional CD-ROM instructions

 Indicates questions and activities that require you to consult your textbook

 Indicates the approximate time required to complete an exercise

Cultural Aspects of Nursing Care

/OℰO **Reading Assignment:** Cultural Aspects of Nursing Care (Chapter 6)

Patients: Piya Jordan, Room 403
Clarence Hughes, Room 404
Pablo Rodriguez, Room 405

Objectives:

1. Describe cultural concepts related to nursing and health care.

2. Identify traditional health habits and beliefs of major ethnic groups in the United States.

3. Explain cultural influences on the interactions of patients and families within the health care system.

4. Discuss considerations for providing culturally sensitive nursing care.

5. Discuss ways in which planning and implementation of nursing interventions can be adapted to a patient's ethnicity.

Exercise 1

Writing Activity

30 minutes

1. Culture is defined as a patterned behavioral response that develops over time. What factors work together to shape culture?

2. Members of a _____ share values that differ from those in their dominant culture.

3. _____ nursing is the integration of culture into all aspects of nursing care.

4. When the nurse is identifying the traits of an ethnic group, what *primary* characteristics should be considered? Select all that apply.

   _____ Race

   _____ Skin color

   _____ Health care practices

   _____ Moral values

   _____ Language

   _____ Cultural origin

   _____ National or geographical origin

5. Which of the following *secondary* characteristics should be given consideration when iden-tifying traits of an ethnic group? Select all that apply.

   _____ A sense of group identity

   _____ Cultural origin

   _____ Attitudes derived from group identity

   _____ Distinctive customs, art, music, literature

   _____ Elements of lifestyles

   _____ Food preferences

6. Although people of differing religions may have contrasting views about illness, their views concerning health are typically very similar.
   a. True
   b. False

7. A patient who reports that he feels his own religious choices are best and superior to those practiced by different groups is demonstrating what behavior?
   a. Monoculturalism
   b. Ethnocentrism
   c. Stereotyping
   d. Biculturalism

8. Using both _____ and _____ communication can help reinforce the information provided to the patient.

9. When administering medications, the nurse must be aware of the influence ethnicity can have on drug therapy. Which of the following factors could potentially affect drug therapy? Select all that apply.

   _____   Environment

   _____   Diet

   _____   Genetic differences

   _____   Nontraditional home remedies

   _____   Patient expectations

10. The beliefs of people of different ethnic groups seem to play a role in the decision of whether or not to place elders in residential facilities. The fact that the majority of residents

    in long-term care facilities are _____ _____ is evidence of these differing beliefs among cultural groups.

11. According to the "hot and cold" theory of illness, which of the following disorders are associated with the entry of cold into the body? Select all that apply.

    _____   Dysentery

    _____   Kidney disease

    _____   Paralysis

    _____   Stomach cramps

    _____   Dental abscesses

12. Caucasians traditionally hold values related to health that include individual

    _____ _____, personal _____, and

    _____.

13. Chinese Americans may exhibit an increased incidence of which of the following diet-related disorders and diseases? Select all that apply.

_____ Heart disease

_____ Cancer of the bowel

_____ Breast cancer

_____ Stomach cancer

_____ Lactose intolerance

_____ Thalassemia deficiency

14. Members of which of the following cultures traditionally consider touching a deceased person to be taboo?
    a. Japanese
    b. Chinese
    c. Navajo
    d. African

Exercise 2

CD-ROM Activity

30 minutes

- Sign in to work at Pacific View Regional Hospital for Period of Care 1. (*Note:* If you are already in the virtual hospital from a previous exercise, click on **Leave the Floor** and then **Restart the Program** to get to the sign-in window.)
- From the Patient List, select Piya Jordan (Room 403), Clarence Hughes (Room 404), and Pablo Rodriguez (Room 405).
- Click on **Get Report** and read the shift report for each of the patients.
- Click on **Go to Nurses' Station**.
- Click on Piya Jordan's room number (**403**) at the bottom of the screen and review the **Initial Observations**.
- Next, click on **Chart** and then on **403** to open Piya Jordan's chart. Review her **History and Physical** and **Nursing Admission**.
- Now repeat the previous two steps with your other two patients, Clarence Hughes and Pablo Rodriguez.

1. Identify the ethnic group to which each patient belongs.

   Piya Jordan: _____

   Clarence Hughes: _____

   Pablo Rodriguez: _____

2. Identify the religious affiliation of each patient.

Piya Jordan: _____

Clarence Hughes: _____

Pablo Rodriguez: _____

3. Religions can be classified as Eastern or Western. Which of the following religions are defined by the textbook as Western? Select all that apply.

_____ Buddhist

_____ American Muslim

_____ Lutheran

_____ Baptist

_____ Roman Catholic

4. Match each of the following beliefs and practices to the corresponding religion with which they are associated.

Belief/Practice	**Religion**
_____ Importance placed on objects such as relics, statues, scapulars, and medals bearing the images of saints	a. Buddhism
_____ May use ritual or contemplation in hopes that the last moments of consciousness may be filled with thoughts worthy of elevation to a higher existence	b. Baptist c. Catholic
_____ Belief in the need for total abstinence from alcohol	
_____ Belief that birth control should be limited to a bstinence or natural family planning	
_____ Belief in reincarnation	

5. Which of the following cultures may embrace the use of healers? Select all that apply.

_____ African Americans

_____ Euro-Americans

_____ Latinos

_____ American Indians

_____ Italians

6. Language may provide a source of anxiety for Piya Jordan during her hospitalization.
   a. True
   b. False

7. Discuss the potential feelings that Piya Jordan may have concerning elders.

8. How do the meanings of the terms *black* and *African American* differ?

9. If Clarence Hughes followed the traditional values of his culture related to illness and health, he would seek early intervention from a physician.
   a. True
   b. False

10. When providing care to Clarence Hughes, the nurse must be knowledgeable about health conditions for which he is at a higher risk of developing because of his ethnic/racial background. Which of the following diseases/disorders does Clarence Hughes have an increased risk for developing?

   _____   Diabetes

   _____   Lactose intolerance

   _____   Hypertension

   _____   Osteoporosis

   _____   Cardiovascular disease

   _____   Cirrhosis

   _____   Sickle cell disease

11. List at least three traditional values and/or behaviors related to health and illness that may be exhibited by African Americans.

12. List several beliefs about health and illness associated with Pablo Rodriguez's cultural, ethnic, and/or religious background. (*Hint:* See Table 6-1 and page 67 in your textbook.)

13. If Pablo Rodriguez were to request anointment by the hospital's priest, the nurse should understand which of the following?
a. Pablo Rodriguez is nearing death.
b. This ritual may be done during times of illness.
c. Pablo Rodriguez has decided to forgo further treatments of his disease.
d. Pablo Rodriguez is feeling better.

Nutrition

Reading Assignment: Nutrition (Chapter 9)

Patient: Piya Jordan, Room 403

Objectives:

1. Explain the functions of the gastrointestinal system in the digestion of food.

2. Describe how food is digested and absorbed.

3. List the functions of each of the six classes of essential nutrients.

4. Define *macronutrient* and *micronutrient*.

5. Identify the food sources of proteins, carbohydrates, and fats.

6. Identify the food sources and possible health benefits of dietary fiber.

7. Identify the food sources of each of the vitamins and minerals.

8. Describe the changes in nutrient needs as an individual ages.

9. Discuss the different types of nutritional support.

Exercise 1

Writing Activity

30 minutes

1. The four main functions of the GI system are _____,

   _____, _____, and _____.

2. Proteins and fiber are nutrients that primarily provide energy.
   a. True
   b. False

3. List the five major components of food.

4. Ingested plant and animal molecules that are used for energy or to synthesize other elements

   from nutritional intake are referred to as _____.

5. An individual's metabolic rate is determined primarily by which of the following? Select all
   that apply.

   _____ Height

   _____ Body surface area

   _____ Body weight

   _____ Race

   _____ Dietary intake

6. Hormones involved in the regulation of blood glucose include which of the following?
   Select all that apply.

   _____ Insulin

   _____ Luteinizing hormone

   _____ Thyroid hormone

   _____ Epinephrine

   _____ Glucocorticoids

   _____ Growth hormone

7. The nurse is providing education to a patient regarding the benefits of a high-fiber diet. Which of the following concepts should be included in the exchange of information? Select all that apply.

_____ Enhanced bowel functioning

_____ Increased energy

_____ Reduced blood cholesterol

_____ Increased rate of glucose absorption

_____ Reduced incidence of colon cancer development

8. A patient has been advised to increase her intake of folic acid in preparation for pregnancy. Which of the following foods should be included in this plan? Select all that apply.

_____ Milk

_____ Eggs

_____ Dried beans

_____ Whole grain products

_____ Yeast

_____ Wheat germ

_____ Leafy green vegetables

9. A patient who has been instructed to begin taking a multivitamin supplement daily questions why this is necessary. Which of the following statements regarding vitamins is correct?
   a. Vitamins are organic substances.
   b. Vitamins provide energy.
   c. Water-soluble vitamins include the B complexes and vitamin C.
   d. Fat-soluble vitamins cannot be stored in the body.

10. Major minerals are responsible for enzyme regulation, _____ balance,

    osmotic pressure, and maintenance of nerve and muscle _____.

11. A nurse is providing care for a patient suspected of being malnourished. Which of the following diagnostic tests will provide the best information to confirm these suspicions?
    a. Serum albumin
    b. Urinalysis
    c. Hematocrit
    d. Complete blood count

12. Fat should account for 30% or less of the daily caloric intake.
    a. True
    b. False

13. A diet high in fat has been associated with the development of _____

_____ , _____ , and _____ .

14. While being seen at the physician's office for a routine physical examination, a patient tells the nurse that he has been hearing a great deal of "hype" about antioxidants. He asks the nurse to explain what they are. Which of the following statements about antioxidants is most accurate?
    a. Antioxidants are plant pigments found in yellow fruits and vegetables.
    b. Antioxidants are hormone-like substances found in whole grains and legumes.
    c. Antioxidants are contained in some foods and are believed to have a role in the prevention of cancer.
    d. Antioxidants are proteins found in onions and wines that are linked to a reduction in the risk for diabetes.

15. A patient attempting to follow a healthy diet asks about the amount of whole grains needed each day. Which of the following is the best response to give to this patient?
    a. "You should try to eat at least 3 ounces of whole grains each day."
    b. "You should eat no more than 4 ounces of whole grains each day."
    c. "You should eat between 2 and 3 ounces of whole grains each day."
    d. "There is no current differentiation between grains and whole grains."

16. A nurse caring for a patient having enteral tube feedings should be aware of potential complications. Which of the following are potential complications associated with enteral tube feedings? Select all that apply.

    _____ Hunger

    _____ Vomiting

    _____ Hyperkalemia

    _____ Hypernatremia

    _____ Diarrhea

Exercise 2

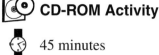 **CD-ROM Activity**

45 minutes

- Sign in to work at Pacific View Regional Hospital for Period of Care 2. (*Note:* If you are already in the virtual hospital from a previous exercise, click on **Leave the Floor** and **Restart the Program** to get to the sign-in window.)
- From the Patient List, select Piya Jordan (Room 403).
- Click on **Get Report** and read the shift report.
- Click on **Go to Nurses' Station** and then on **Chart**.
- Click on **403** to view Piya Jordan's chart.
- Click on and review the **History and Physical** and **Nursing Admission**.

1. List Piya Jordan's identified health care concerns.

2. Piya Jordan's weight is _____ pounds (_____ kg), and she is _____ inches tall.

3. Piya Jordan reports a recent weight loss of _____ pounds.

4. Based on her age and sedentary lifestyle, how many calories per day does Piya Jordan require?
   a. 1200
   b. 1500
   c. 1600
   d. 2200

→ • Click on and review the **Laboratory Reports** in Piya Jordan's chart.

5. Piya Jordan's hematocrit levels range between _____% and _____%.

6. Normal hematocrit levels for women are between _____% and _____%.

7. Which of the following statements concerning hematocrit levels are correct? Select all that apply.

_____ The hematocrit level indicates the body's protein level.

_____ Hematocrit is a measurement of the body's iron status.

_____ Hematocrit levels are the same for both men and women.

_____ Surgical intervention can alter the body's hematocrit levels.

_____ Dehydration is associated with a decrease in hematocrit.

8. Urine specific gravity is normally between _____ and _____.

9. Piya Jordan's urine specific gravity is _____.

10. Indicate whether each of following statements is true or false.

a. _____ A reduced urine specific gravity is indicative of hypovolemia.

b. _____ Based on a review of Piya Jordan's laboratory findings, the mean corpuscular volume indicates the presence of anemia.

→ • Click on and review the **Physician's Notes** and **Physician's Orders**.

11. Which of the following events can increase the body's nutritional needs? Select all that apply.

_____ Infection

_____ Fever

_____ Trauma

_____ Stress

_____ Rest

12. What diet has been ordered for Piya Jordan?

13. What nutrition is being provided to Piya Jordan during this stage of her recovery?

14. Over the course of a 24-hour day, Piya Jordan will receive _____ mL of the D$_5$NS infusion.

15. The amount and type of IV fluids being provided to Piya Jordan are adequate to prevent dehydration and provide adequate nutrition.
    a. True
    b. False

16. Piya Jordan's prescribed intravenous fluids can best be described as:
    a. a Ringer's solution.
    b. a source of total parenteral nutrition.
    c. a hypotonic dextrose solution.
    d. an isotonic saline solution.
    e. a hypertonic dextrose solution.

17. Which of the following statements best explains the intended action of Piya Jordan's ordered intravenous solution (D$_5$NS)?
    a. Mimics electrolyte concentration of blood
    b. Often used as a volume expander
    c. Provides energy and nutrients for cellular function and repair
    d. Expands extracellular fluid without changing osmolality

18. Piya Jordan's IV site must be assessed frequently. The presence of complications can be identified by manifestations at the site and by observations of the patient. Match each of the following complications with the corresponding clinical manifestation.

Complication	Clinical Manifestation
_____ Infiltration	a. Heat, pain, redness, and edema
_____ Phlebitis	b. Heat, pain, redness, edema, and possible fever and sepsis
_____ Infection	
_____ Air embolism	c. Fluid that will not flow by gravity; site that is edematous, blanched, painful, and cold
_____ Allergic reaction	d. Rash, redness, and itching
_____ Circulatory overload	e. Cyanosis, tachycardia, and decreased blood pressure
	f. Dyspnea, cough, cyanosis, and jugular vein distention

19. After _____ days without oral nutrition, enteral methods may be indicated.

20. A nasogastric (NG) tube may be used for which of the following reasons? Select all that apply.

_____ Decompression—removal of secretions and gases from the GI tract

_____ Feeding—instillation of liquid supplements or feedings into the stomach

_____ Compression—internal application of pressure by means of an inflated balloon to prevent internal GI hemorrhage

_____ Evacuation—reduction of intestinal stool contents

_____ Lavage—irrigation of stomach; used in cases of active bleeding, poisoning, or gastric dilation

21. The nurse is planning to clean Piya Jordan's nostril where the NG tube is placed. Which of the following solutions is most appropriate for use?
   a. Alcohol-based solution
   b. Mild soap and water
   c. Hydrogen peroxide
   d. Water-soluble lubricant

22. When monitoring Piya Jordan's NG output, which of the following findings may indicate fluid volume deficits? Select all that apply.

_____ Hypotension

_____ Pulse of more than 20 beats per minute above the baseline values

_____ Hypertension

_____ Urine production of less than 50 mL/hr for 2 or more consecutive hours

_____ Confusion

23. Output totals of _____ mL or greater from the NG tube warrant notification of the physician.

24. Use the MyPyramid food guidance system to match each of the following food groups with the recommended daily servings for a 3000-calorie-per-day diet. (*Hint:* See page 111 in your textbook.)

Food Group		Number of Servings
_____	Grains	a. 3 cups per day
_____	Vegetables	b. 10 ounces per day
_____	Fruits	c. 7 ounces per day
_____	Milk	d. 2½ cups per day
_____	Meats and beans	e. 4 cups per day

Developmental Processes and the Older Adult

👓 **Reading Assignment:** Developmental Processes (Chapter 10)
The Older Patient (Chapter 11)

Patient: Clarence Hughes, Room 404

Objectives:

1. List the developmental tasks for successful adulthood.

2. Identify the health problems specific to the adult age groups.

3. Discuss the health care needs of young, middle, and older adults.

4. Describe the roles of the gerontological nurse.

5. Describe modifications needed for activities of daily living.

6. Determine the extent to which selected myths and stereotypes about older adults are factual.

7. Describe biological, physiological, and psychosocial factors associated with aging.

8. Explain why drug adjustments may be needed for older persons.

Exercise 1

Writing Activity

30 minutes

1. Identify the developmental tasks that must be achieved by young adults. Select all that apply.

   _____ Discover new satisfaction with a mate or significant other

   _____ Begin preparation for retirement

   _____ Establish independence

   _____ Become established in a vocation or profession that provides personal satisfaction, economic independence, and a sense of purpose

   _____ Maintain a home and manage a time schedule and life stresses

2. The physiological development of a living being and the qualitative changes seen in the body are known as _____.

3. _____ is the progression of behavioral changes that involve the acquisition of appropriate cognitive, linguistic, and psychosocial skills.

4. The study of aging is known as _____.

5. _____ is a stereotype, prejudice, or discrimination against people, especially older adults, based on their age.

6. Some degree of intellectual decline is a normal part of aging.
   a. True
   b. False

7. Identify the stages of adulthood and include the age range for each stage.

8. A student nurse is preparing a presentation concerning the "sandwich generation." Which of the following statements about this concept is correct?
   a. The name is derived from the amount of fast food consumed during this generation.
   b. Members of the sandwich generation include school-age children.
   c. Adults in their middle years are members of this category.
   d. Elder adults are members of the sandwich generation.

9. If a nurse is performing an assessment on a middle adult patient, which of the following must be included to determine successful completion of the appropriate developmental tasks?
   a. Assess for the presence of meaningful, intimate relationships
   b. Assess for signs of depression, such as excessive sleeping and decreased appetite
   c. Ask the patient if he or she feels lonely
   d. Assess for the presence of parental support systems

10. Which of the following is the major cause of death for patients between the ages of 39 and 45?
   a. Suicide
   b. Homicide
   c. Cancer
   d. Accidents

11. A middle-age female patient asks about her risk for osteoporosis during this period in her life. Which of the following is the best response by the nurse?
   a. Osteoporosis is not a concern until late adulthood.
   b. Osteoporosis is only an issue for underweight women.
   c. Osteoporosis is a greater concern for young women of childbearing age.
   d. It is too late to prevent osteoporosis-related complications.
   e. Osteoporosis is a concern for women in middle age.

12. The leading cause of death for older adults is:
   a. heart disease.
   b. unintentional injuries.
   c. AIDS.
   d. bone cancer.

13. Which of the following refers to the functional capabilities of various organ systems in the body?
   a. Biologic age
   b. Psychological age
   c. Social age
   d. Chronological age

14. When providing health education to a preteen female, the nurse should incorporate which of the following characteristics into the teaching?
   a. The rate of physical growth exceeds the rate of cognitive development.
   b. If the child had begun to demonstrate physical changes, she is considered to be an adolescent.
   c. Some girls in this age group may begin to demonstrate the changes associated with puberty.
   d. The rate of physical growth exceeds the rate of psychosocial development.

8. Which of the following statements concerning the use of medications in older adults are true? Select all that apply.

_____ On average, the older adult takes up to seven prescription medications.

_____ Laxatives and vitamin supplements are commonly used medications among older adults.

_____ The average older adult is currently taking only two prescription medications.

_____ The use of multiple drugs will enhance the therapeutic benefits of the medications taken.

_____ Using more than one pharmacy to fill prescriptions will increase risk factors associated with polypharmacy.

_____ The body's ability to absorb, transport, and eliminate mediations is increased with age.

→ • Click on **Return to Room 404**.
 • Click on the **Drug** icon in the lower left corner.
 • Review the information for each of the medications ordered for Clarence Hughes.

9. Which of the prescribed medications listed below have special life span considerations listed for older adults? Select all that apply.

_____ Celecoxib

_____ Timolol maleate

_____ Docusate sodium

_____ Pilocarpine 1% ophthalmic solution

_____ Enoxaparin

_____ Promethazine hydrochloride

_____ Magnesium hydroxide

_____ Aluminum hydroxide with magnesium and simethicone

_____ Bisacodyl

10. Which of the following are manifestations associated with adverse drug reactions in the older adult? Select all that apply.

_____ Restlessness

_____ Falls

_____ Excitability

_____ Depression

_____ Altered mental states

_____ Diarrhea

_____ Urinary incontinence

11. Match each of the following drug classifications with its adverse reaction associated with aging.

Drug Classification	**Adverse Reaction**
_____ Antibiotics	a. Drowsiness
_____ Antidepressants	b. Nephrotoxicity
_____ Antipsychotics	c. Confusion
_____ Diuretics	d. Hypokalemia
_____ Sedatives/hypnotics	e. Sedation

12. Identify several factors that can reduce medication-related complications in the elderly patient.

Inflammation, Infection, and Immunity

Reading Assignment: Inflammation, Infection, and Immunity (Chapter 13)

Patient: Harry George, Room 401

Objectives:

1. Describe physical and chemical barriers to infection.

2. Describe how inflammatory changes act as bodily defense mechanisms.

3. Identify the signs and symptoms of inflammation.

4. Discuss the process of repair and healing.

5. Differentiate between infection and inflammation.

6. Describe the ways that infections are transmitted.

7. Identify the signs and symptoms of infection.

8. Compare community-acquired and nosocomial infections.

9. Discuss the nursing care of patients with infections.

Exercise 1

Writing Activity

30 minutes

1. The body's first lines of defense are the _____ and

   _____ _____.

2. Match each of the following cell types with its role in immunity.

   Cell Type   **Role**

   _____ Neutrophils   a. Increase the body's immune response

   _____ Monocytes   b. Fight bacterial infections

   _____ Eosinophils   c. Initiate the inflammatory response and release
                                       histamine

   _____ Basophils
                                    d. Produce antibodies

   _____ B lymphocytes
                                    e. Ingest foreign antigens

   _____ T lymphocytes
                                    f. Fight parasitic infections and demonstrate an
                                       increase during allergic reactions

3. List the actions of the inflammatory process in order of occurrence.

   Action   **Order of Occurrence**

   _____ Chemical mediation   a. First

   _____ Hemodynamic change   b. Second

   _____ Antiinflammation hormones released c. Third

   _____ Increased capillary permeability   d. Fourth

4. A patient has been diagnosed with ringworm infection. Based on your knowledge, you
   recognize that this patient has a:
   a. viral infection.
   b. bacterial infection.
   c. protozoan infection.
   d. fungal infection.

5. If a patient has been diagnosed with a sexually transmitted disease, which of the following
   modes of transfer has taken place?
   a. Direct contact
   b. Indirect contact
   c. Multifocal contact
   d. Common vehicle transmission

6. A nurse working in a physician's office should recognize that which of the following diseases and/or infections are considered reportable? Select all that apply.

   _____ Herpes simplex

   _____ Gonorrhea

   _____ Candidiasis

   _____ Rubella

   _____ Tetanus

7. _____ - _____ infections are acquired in day-to-day contact with the public.

8. Infections that occur within a health care facility are known as _____

   _____.

9. Indicate whether each of the following statements is true or false.

   a. _____ Medication administration requires the use of sterile technique.

   b. _____ The most effective tool in the prevention of cross-contamination is hand-washing.

10. Match each of the following disorders with the correct method of precaution. (*Note:* Some methods of precaution will be used more than once.)

Disease	**Method of Precaution**
_____ Measles	a. Airborne precautions
_____ Varicella	b. Droplet precautions
_____ Mumps	c. Contact precautions
_____ Tuberculosis	
_____ *Clostridium difficile* infection	
_____ Scabies	
_____ Pediculosis	
_____ Influenza	

11. Discuss the difference between antigens and antibodies.

12. Innate immunity is present in the body at birth.
    a. True
    b. False

Exercise 2

 CD-ROM Activity

45 minutes

- Sign in to work at Pacific View Regional Hospital for Period of Care 1. (*Note:* If you are already in the virtual hospital from a previous exercise, click on **Leave the Floor** and then **Restart the Program** to get to the sign-in window.)
- From the Patient List, select Harry George (Room 401).
- Click on **Get Report** and read the shift report.
- Click on **Go to Nurses' Station**.
- Click on **Chart** and then on **401**.
- Click on and review the **Nursing Admission** and **History and Physical**.

1. What were the chief complaints voiced by Harry George on his arrival to the Emergency Department?

2. What medical diagnoses are listed on the History and Physical?

→ • Click on and review the **Laboratory Reports**.

3. Harry George has been diagnosed with a viral infection.
   a. True
   b. False

4. The physician has ordered an erythrocyte sedimentation rate drawn. Which of the following statements best describes this test?
   a. The erythrocyte sedimentation rate is suppressed in the presence of inflammation.
   b. An infectious process will reduce the sedimentation rate.
   c. The erythrocyte sedimentation rate is elevated in the presence of inflammation.
   d. The erythrocyte sedimentation rate is naturally suppressed in alcohol-dependent patients.

5. Which of the following tests will be ordered to confirm the presence of the infection in Harry George? Select all that apply.

   _____ Complete blood cell count

   _____ Culture and sensitivity of wound

   _____ Urinalysis

   _____ MRI

   _____ Folic acid level

   _____ Blood alcohol level

6. Harry George's white blood cell count has ranged from _____ on Monday to _____ on Tuesday.

7. The normal range for the white blood cell count is:
   a. 2,000-4,500.
   b. 4,000-7,500.
   c. 4,400-11,000.
   d. 10,000-12,000.

8. The pathogen identified as the causative agent in Harry George's infection is

   _____ _____.

9. The causative agent in Harry George's infection can be further identified as:
   a. bacterial.
   b. fungal.
   c. protozoan.
   d. rickettsiae.
   e. parasitic.

10. It is a legal requirement that Harry George's infection be reported to the appropriate public health officials.
    a. True
    b. False

→ • Click on **Return to Nurses' Station**; then click on **401**.
 • Review the **Initial Observations**.
 • Click on **Patient Care** and then on **Physical Assessment**.
 • Complete a head-to-toe systems assessment.

11. When the nurse is preparing to care for Harry George, which of the following precautions is warranted?
 a. Enteric precautions
 b. Droplet precautions
 c. Reverse isolation
 d. Airborne precautions
 e. Standard precautions
 f. Universal precautions

12. Which of the following will place Harry George at the greatest risk for developing a nosocomial infection?
 a. Indwelling Foley catheter
 b. Increasing pain
 c. History of alcohol abuse
 d. Homelessness

13. What findings in Harry George's lower extremities support the presence of an infection?

14. Which of the following stages of antiinflammatory response is most likely being demonstrated in Harry George's assessment?
 a. Stage 1
 b. Stage 2
 c. Stage 3
 d. Stage 4

15. Harry George's wound has redness, warmth, and swelling. This is representative of the

 _____ changes in the inflammatory process.

→ • Click on **MAR** and then on **401**.
 • Review Harry George's ordered medications. (*Hint:* If necessary, refer to the Drug Guide for assistance.)

16. What medications have been ordered to manage Harry George's infection?

17. Which of the following assessments related to Harry George's IV therapy are indicated as a result of the prescribed gentamicin? Select all that apply.

_____ Induration

_____ Heat along vein

_____ Redness surrounding IV site

_____ Presence of red streaks

_____ Pain

18. Which of the following manifestations is consistent with a serious complication of the administration of gentamicin?
a. Nausea
b. Genital pruritis
c. Lethargy
d. Diarrhea

Pain Management

Reading Assignment: Pain Management (Chapter 15)

Patients: Harry George, Room 401
Pablo Rodriguez, Room 405

Objectives:

1. Define *pain*.

2. Explain the physiologic basis for pain.

3. Identify situations in which patients are likely to experience pain.

4. Explain the relationships between a patient's pain and past pain experiences, anticipation, culture, anxiety, and/or activity.

5. Identify differences in the duration of acute and chronic pain and discuss patient responses to each.

6. Explain the special needs of the older adult patient with pain.

7. List the data to be collected in assessing pain.

8. Describe the nursing care of patients receiving opioid and nonopioid analgesics for pain.

9. List the factors that should be considered when pain is not relieved with analgesic medications.

Exercise 1

 Writing Activity

🕐 30 minutes

1. _____ are pain receptors located in the muscles, tendons, subcutaneous tissue, and the skin.

2. _____ are the body's natural opioid-like substances that block the transmission of painful impulses to the brain.

3. A _____ is an inactive substance used in research or clinical practice to determine the effects of a legitimate drug or treatment.

4. Which of the following are factors that can increase the body's endorphin levels? Select all that apply.

_____ Age

_____ Gender

_____ Brief stress

_____ Pain

_____ Laughter

_____ Exercise

_____ Beliefs about pain

5. Identify several physical factors that can affect a patient's perception of pain.

6. Indicate whether each of the following statements is true or false.

a. _____ Gender can affect an individual's pain threshold and tolerance.

b. _____ While caring for a patient who has recently been medicated for complaints of pain, it is appropriate for the nurse to ask the nursing assistant to recheck the patient's level of pain.

7. The nurse is planning to use heat to manage a patient's pain. Which of the following statements concerning the use of heat therapy are correct? Select all that apply.

_____ Heat therapy may be alternated with cold therapy.

_____ Heat therapy is contraindicated in patients with peripheral vascular disease.

_____ Heat therapy should be limited to 30 minutes per application.

_____ Heat applications may be moist or dry.

_____ Heat is a safe, effective means to manage pain related to a malignant tumor.

8. A nurse is preparing to provide an inservice on the use of alternative treatments for pain. Which of the following concepts are correct and may be included in the presentation? Select all that apply.

_____ Chiropractic treatments may increase patient depression.

_____ Massage therapy may lessen anxiety and depression.

_____ Music therapy has no untoward side effects.

_____ Unwillingness to be touched may hinder the success of massage therapy.

_____ Music therapy is an expensive alternative for pain management.

9. A _____ unit involves the application of external electrical stimulation of the skin and underlying tissues through electrodes attached to the skin.

10. While caring for a patient, a nurse notes the presence of agitation, insomnia, diarrhea, and sweating after requests for "stronger" analgesics are refused by the physician. Which of the following is being demonstrated by the patient?
    a. The patient has developed a tolerance to all analgesics.
    b. The patient has developed psychological dependence.
    c. The patient is an alcoholic and needs a drink.
    d. The patient has developed physiological dependence.

11. Match each of the following pain characteristics with the type of pain it is most likely to be associated with.

Characteristic	**Type of Pain**
_____ Usually responds to commonly prescribed medical and nursing interventions	a. Acute pain
_____ May not be associated with an identified injury or event	b. Chronic pain
_____ Consists of discomfort lasting 1-2 months	
_____ Includes evidence of tissue damage	
_____ May not be reported	

12. A patient who has recently undergone surgery questions the use of narcotic analgesics and is concerned about becoming "hooked." Which of the following statements by the nurse is most therapeutic?
    a. "You should avoid the use of narcotics after the first postoperative day to reduce the incidence of addiction."
    b. "Addiction is an unfortunate but common event during the postoperative period."
    c. "Taking the ordered pain medicine every 6 hours will reduce the incidence of becoming addicted."
    d. "Becoming addicted to pain medication after short-term use is uncommon."
    e. "Do you have a history of alcohol or drug dependence?"

13. Which of the following are associated with undertreatment of pain by health care providers? Select all that apply.

    _____ Concerns about the cost of medications prescribed

    _____ Inadequate information about the drugs ordered

    _____ Anxiety about potential patient injuries suffered while being medicated

    _____ Laziness of the health care provider

    _____ Concerns about fostering addiction

14. Opioid analgesics and nonopioid analgesics can be administered together.
    a. True
    b. False

15. When administering nonopioid analgesics to a patient who has congestive heart failure, the nurse should perform what assessment to monitor for the presence of related adverse reactions?
    a. Intake and output
    b. Respiratory rate
    c. Temperature
    d. The presence of cramping and diarrhea
    e. The onset of a superinfection

Exercise 2

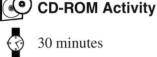 **CD-ROM Activity**

 30 minutes

- Sign in to work at Pacific View Regional Hospital for Period of Care 2. (*Note:* If you are already in the virtual hospital from a previous exercise, click on **Leave the Floor** and then **Restart the Program** to get to the sign-in window.)
- From the Patient List, select Harry George (Room 401).
- Click on **Get Report** and read the shift report.
- Click on **Go to Nurses' Station** and then on **401**.
- Click on and review the **Clinical Alerts**.

1. Harry George is reporting pain at a level of _____ on a _____-point scale.

2. The type of scale being used to assess Harry George's pain is known as a:
   a. visual analogue scale.
   b. numerical rating scale.
   c. verbal descriptor scale.
   d. linear pain continuum scale.

➡ • Click on **Chart** and then on **401**.
- Click on and review the **Nursing Admission** and **History and Physical**.

3. What are Harry George's medical diagnoses?

➡ • Click on **Return to Room 401**.
- Click on **MAR** and then on tab **401**.
- Review Harry George's ordered medications.

4. According to the nurse's entry on the MAR, Harry George may be remedicated for complaints of pain at _____.

5. How long after hydromorphone hydrochloride is administered to Harry George should interventions be performed to ensure maximum effectiveness of the drug? (*Hint:* Refer to the Drug Guide as necessary.)
   a. 10 minutes
   b. 15-30 minutes
   c. 30-60 minutes
   d. 2 hours
   e. 3 hours

6. If the administration route of the hydromorphone hydrochloride is changed to PO, what dosage of medication can be anticipated, assuming that Harry George's pain remains at the same level?
   a. 2 mg
   b. 7.5 mg
   c. 4 mg
   d. The calculation cannot be determined.

7. Opioid analgesic medications may be one of two types. Which of the following medications are classified as opioid agonists? Select all that apply.

   _____ Codeine

   _____ Methadone

   _____ Buprenorphine (Buprenex)

   _____ Nalbuphine (Nubain)

   _____ Hydromorphone (Dilaudid)

   _____ Meperidine (Demerol)

8. Which of the following methods for administering analgesics will be most effective for Harry George: around the clock (ATC) or as needed (PRN)? Why?

9. Indicate whether each of the following statements is true or false.

   a. _____ Hydromorphone has a ceiling effect on analgesia.

   b. _____ Harry George's physician has ordered his analgesics to be given every 3 hours prn. The nurse may administer them ATC if the q3h schedule is adhered to.

10. Use the Sedation Scale to evaluate Harry George's current status. Which of the following best identifies his status during this period of care?
    a. S
    b. 1
    c. 2
    d. 3
    e. 4

11. When developing a plan of care for Harry George, the nurse knows that which of the following nursing diagnoses is most appropriate and has the highest priority?
    a. Activity intolerance
    b. Ineffective role performance
    c. Ineffective coping
    d. Hopelessness
    e. Disturbed body image
    f. Acute pain

Exercise 3

CD-ROM Activity

30 minutes

- Sign in to work at Pacific View Regional Hospital for Period of Care 2. (*Note:* If you are already in the virtual hospital from a previous exercise, click on **Leave the Floor** and then **Restart the Program** to get to the sign-in window.)
- From the Patient List, select Pablo Rodriguez (Room 405).
- Click on **Get Report** and read the shift report.
- Click on **Go to Nurses' Station** and then on **405**.
- Click on and review the **Clinical Alerts**.

1. Presently, Pablo Rodriguez is reporting a pain level of _____ on a 10-point scale.

- Click on **Chart** and then on **405**.
- Click on and review the **Nursing Admission** and **History and Physical**.

2. What are Pablo Rodriguez's medical diagnoses?

- Click on **Return to Room 405**.
- Click on **Patient Care** and then on **Physical Assessment** to complete a head-to-toe assessment of Pablo Rodriguez.

3. Based on your assessment, which of the following are sources of discomfort for Pablo Rodriguez? Select all that apply.

_____ Condition of the oral cavity

_____ Constipation

_____ Ability to urinate

_____ Breathing

_____ Subcutaneous nodules

_____ Lymph nodes in the neck

→ • Click on **EPR** and then on **Login**.
• Select **405** as the patient and **Vital Signs** as the category.
• Review the information concerning Pablo Rodriguez's pain during this hospitalization.

4. During this hospitalization, the range of reported pain levels for Pablo Rodriguez has been

between _____ and _____.

5. Which of the following characteristics are used to describe Pablo Rodriguez's pain on Wednesday? Select all that apply.

_____ Aching

_____ Burning

_____ Chronic

_____ Dull

_____ Electric

_____ Intermittent

_____ Internal

_____ Sharp

_____ Shooting

→ • Click on **Exit EPR**.
• Click on **MAR** and then on tab **405**.
• Review Pablo Rodriguez's ordered medications.

6. Match each of Pablo Rodriguez's ordered medications with its correct classification.

Medication	Classification
_____ Morphine sulfate	a. Antiemetic; blocks serotonin
_____ Metoclopramide hydrochloride	b. Ammonia detoxicant
_____ Mineral oil	c. Schedule II narcotic analgesic
_____ Zolpidem tartrate	d. Stool softener
_____ Dexamethasone	e. Schedule IV hypnotic
_____ Senna	f. Antiemetic; reduces esophageal reflux
_____ Lactulose	g. Laxative
_____ Ondansetron hydrochloride	h. Corticosteroid

7. What is the rationale for ordering two analgesics to manage Pablo Rodriguez's pain?
   a. Providing the IV push medication will reduce his dependence on the PCA pump.
   b. Having multiple analgesic orders will allow him to choose which is preferred.
   c. This is a standard order.
   d. Having the two medications provides a means to manage breakthrough pain.

8. Opioids have been ordered to manage Pablo Rodriguez's pain. Which of the following best describes the manner in which these medications work?
   a. Interfere with the relay of the pain signal across the synapse
   b. Inhibit prostaglandin synthesis
   c. Reduce serotonin availability to reduce pain occurrence
   d. Prevent and block the generation of the pain signals sent

9. Identify the potential side effects associated with opioid use. Select all that apply.

   _____ Diarrhea

   _____ Constipation

   _____ Drowsiness

   _____ Nausea

   _____ Hypertension

   _____ Bradycardia

   _____ Diaphoresis

10. What nonpharmacological interventions can be used to manage Pablo Rodriguez's pain?

11. The MAR reports that Pablo Rodriguez has a continuous PCA pump with morphine sulfate PCA 1 mg/mL, 0.5 mg every 10 min/12 mg in 4-hour lockout. What is the maximum amount of morphine that may be delivered by the PCA pump in a 4-hour period?
    a. 10 mg
    b. 12 mg
    c. 6 mg
    d. 24 mg

12. Indicate whether each of the following statements is true or false.

    a. _____ Meperidine (Demerol) will likely be a suitable alternative for the management of Pablo Rodriguez's pain.

    b. _____ Dosages of morphine sulfate should be held if the patient's respirations are less than 14 per minute.

Surgical Care

Reading Assignment: Surgical Care (Chapter 17)

Patients: Piya Jordan, Room 403

Objectives:

1. State the purpose of each type of surgery: diagnostic, exploratory, curative, palliative, and cosmetic.

2. List data to be included in the nursing assessment of the preoperative patient.

3. Assist in identifying the nursing diagnoses, goals, outcome criteria, and interventions during the preoperative phase of the surgical experience.

4. Outline a preoperative teaching plan.

5. List the responsibilities for each member of the surgical team.

6. Explain the nursing implications for each type of anesthesia.

7. Explain how the nurse can help prevent postoperative complications.

8. List data to be included in the nursing assessment of the postoperative patient.

9. Identify nursing diagnoses, goals, outcome criteria, and interventions for the postoperative patient.

10. Explain patient needs to be considered in discharge teaching.

Exercise 1

Writing Activity

30 minutes

1. Nurses who care for patients before, during, and after surgery are called

   _____ nurses.

2. Match each of the following types of surgery with its correct definition.

Type of Surgery	Definition
_____ Diagnostic	a. Relieves symptoms or improves function without providing a solution to the basic problem
_____ Exploratory	b. Used to remove and study tissue to make a diagnosis
_____ Curative	
_____ Palliative	c. Performed to correct defects that affect appearance
_____ Cosmetic	d. Used to diagnose and determine the extent of a disease process
	e. Used to remove diseased tissue or to correct defects

3. Identify several variables that can affect surgical outcomes.

4. While preparing a patient for surgery, the nurse presents the surgical consent for the patient's signature. The patient reports he does not understand what the physician told him about the rationale for the procedure. Which of the following responses by the nurse is most appropriate?
   a. "This is just a formality. You can sign anyway."
   b. "Let me explain the procedure so that you can sign."
   c. "I will contact your physician so that you can ask for clarification."
   d. "You won't be able to get better without this surgery."

5. Which of the following patients are able to provide informed consent for surgery? Select all that apply.

   _____ A 101-year-old male

   _____ A married 17-year-old female

   _____ A 21-year-old female who has received preoperative medications

   _____ A 17-year-old male

   _____ A confused 34-year-old male

6. A patient is admitted to the clinical facility for an unexpected surgery. During the data collection, the nurse determines the patient had toast and hot tea earlier in the day. How much fasting time is typically required prior to surgery after ingesting a meal of this type?
   a. 2 hours
   b. 4 hours
   c. 6 hours
   d. 8 hours
   e. Overnight

7. Match each of the following types of anesthesia with its correct definition.

   Anesthesia

   _____ Local

   _____ General

   _____ Regional

   _____ Nerve block

   _____ Spinal

   Definition

   a. Produced by inhalation or injection of anesthetic drugs into the bloodstream; causing a loss of all sensation and consciousness

   b. Injection of an agent into vessels; producing a lack of sensation over a specific body area

   c. The temporary loss of feeling as a result of the inhibition of nerve endings in a specific part of the body

   d. Known as subarachnoid block; used for surgical procedures on the lower abdomen, perineum, and lower extremities

   e. The instillation of medication into or around the nerves to block the transmission of nerve impulses in a particular area or region

8. After administering spinal anesthesia, keeping the patient _____ may reduce the risk for developing a postprocedural headache.

9. The use of multiple drugs to manage a patient's anesthesia is referred to as

   _____ _____.

10. During a surgical procedure, the physician reports that the patient is demonstrating signs consistent with malignant hyperthermia. Which of the following manifestations are consistent with this phenomenon? Select all that apply.

_____ Increasing systolic blood pressure

_____ A reduction in diastolic blood pressure

_____ Tachycardia

_____ Muscle rigidity

_____ Cyanosis

_____ Increasing body temperature

11. After a patient undergoes conscious sedation, which of the following criteria must be met prior to discharge? Select all that apply.

_____ Stable vital signs

_____ Intact motor function

_____ Tolerating ordered diet

_____ Ability to void

_____ Patent airway

12. _____ refers to the reopening of a surgical wound.

13. The protrusion of organs from an open wound is known as _____.

14. Match each of the following types of wound drainage with its corresponding characteristics.

Drainage Type	Characteristic
_____ Serous	a. Pink, watery drainage consisting of plasma and red blood cells
_____ Sanguineous	b. Clear, watery plasma drainage
_____ Serosanguineous	c. A protein-rich drainage, which is the result of the liquefaction of necrotic tissue
_____ Purulent	d. Red drainage

15. A patient has a surgical wound in which a considerable amount of tissue was lost. The wound has healed with granulation tissue and epithelization. What type of healing has this patient demonstrated?
a. Primary intention
b. Secondary intention
c. Tertiary intention
d. Mixed intention

16. Indicate whether each of the following statements is true or false.

   a. _____ A patient who had surgery 36 hours ago and currently has a temperature of 100.4 is demonstrating the onset of an infection.

   b. _____ Older patients do not develop high fevers in the presence of an infection during the postoperative period.

17. If a surgical patient has a history of diabetes, which of the following events associated with the condition may increase the risk for the development of complications? Select all that apply.

   _____ Impaired tissue perfusion

   _____ Increased red blood cell count

   _____ Inhibition of leukocyte activity

   _____ Reduced platelet count

   _____ Slowed inflammatory response

Exercise 2

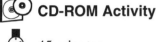 **CD-ROM Activity**

45 minutes

• Sign in to work at Pacific View Regional Hospital for Period of Care 1. (*Note:* If you are already in the virtual hospital from a previous exercise, click on **Leave the Floor** and then **Restart the Program** to get to the sign-in window.)
• From the Patient List, select Piya Jordan (Room 403).
• Click on **Get Report** and read the shift report.
• Click on **Go to Nurses' Station**.
• Click on **Chart** and then on **403**.
• Click on and review the **Nursing Admission**.

   1. Why has Piya Jordan come to the hospital?

   2. How old is Piya Jordan?

3. Why do older patients have additional risks associated with surgery?

4. Piya Jordan's past medical history reflects disorders in which of the following body systems? Select all that apply.

_____ Pulmonary

_____ Cardiovascular

_____ Renal

_____ Neurologic

_____ Metabolic

_____ Integumentary

_____ Gastrointestinal

_____ Musculoskeletal

→ • Click on and review the **Surgical Reports** and **Physician's Notes**.

5. What surgical procedure was performed on Piya Jordan?

6. Which of the following surgical types describes the procedures performed on Piya Jordan? Select all that apply.

_____ Diagnostic

_____ Ablative

_____ Palliative

_____ Constructive

_____ Reconstructive

_____ Transplant

7. Piya Jordan had _____ anesthesia.

➤ • Click on and review the **Laboratory Reports** and **Diagnostic Reports**.

8. Which of the following laboratory tests were performed on Piya Jordan during the preoperative phase? Select all that apply.

_____ Complete blood count

_____ Urinalysis

_____ Serum cholesterol levels

_____ Type and crossmatch

_____ Arterial blood gases

_____ Electrolyte panel

9. Laboratory testing completed during Piya Jordan's preoperative period reflected some abnormal values. Which of the following laboratory values were abnormal during the preoperative phase? Select all that apply.

_____ RBC

_____ INR

_____ Potassium

_____ Sodium

_____ Hemoglobin

_____ Hematocrit

_____ Creatinine

_____ PT

10. For which of the following complications is Piya Jordan at risk because of her INR reading?
   a. Urinary retention
   b. Pneumonia
   c. Paralytic ileus
   d. Hemorrhage

11. Which of the following diagnostic tests were used to confirm the presence of an abdominal mass in Piya Jordan? Select all that apply.

_____ Chest x-ray

_____ KUB

_____ IVP

_____ Colonoscopy

_____ CT scan of abdomen

12. Piya Jordan has drug allergies that may influence the medications prescribed by the physician in both the preoperative and postoperative phases.
    a. True
    b. False

13. During the preoperative period, Piya Jordan received _____ as a preoperative sedative. This medication also has amnesic effects.

14. During the preoperative period, Piya Jordan received _____ as a prophylactic antibiotic.

15. During the preoperative period, the physician ordered the administration of phytonadione 10 mg subQ. Why was this medication administered?

16. Identify the intervention used to prepare Piya Jordan's bowel for the operative procedure.
    a. Mineral oil enema
    b. Fleet enema
    c. Soap suds enema
    d. Oil retention enema
    e. No enema was administered because of the presence of the abdominal mass.

17. Piya Jordan's home medications, digoxin and warfarin, can increase the effects of general anesthesia. (*Hint:* See page 249 in your textbook.)
    a. True
    b. False

18. During the surgical procedure, which of the following responsibilities are included in the role of the circulating nurse? Select all that apply.

_____ Patient assessment

_____ Setting up the surgical room

_____ Handling the instruments within the sterile field

_____ Providing assistance with patient positioning

_____ Monitoring for the use of aseptic technique

_____ Maintaining patient safety

19. Piya Jordan has an indwelling Foley catheter. Which of the following best explains the rationale for its insertion prior to surgery?
    a. The Foley catheter will allow for close monitoring of urinary output.
    b. Having a Foley catheter will allow the patient to rest instead of needing to walk to the bathroom or commode.
    c. The Foley catheter will reduce the occurrence of urinary tract infections.
    d. The Foley catheter reduces the size of the bladder and reduces the chance for injury during the surgical procedure.

20. Piya Jordan has a Jackson-Pratt drain. Which of the following statements about this device are correct? Select all that apply.

_____ It was placed in Piya Jordan's incision while she was in the PACU.

_____ It will reduce fluid accumulation between surfaces of the wound.

_____ It is a small, pliable flat latex tube used to promote drainage.

_____ It is a closed drainage system.

_____ It is an open drainage system.

_____ It has a cartridge.

_____ It has a bulb.

• Click on **Return to Nurses' Station**.
• Click on **403** at the bottom of the screen.
• Review the **Initial Observations**.
• Click on **Patient Care** and then on **Physical Assessment** to perform a systems assessment.

21. When performing an assessment of Piya Jordan's incision, the nurse should include which of the following? Select all that apply.

_____ Approximation of the sutures

_____ Color of tissue surrounding the incision

_____ The presence of drainage from the incision

_____ Total number of sutures

_____ Odor of the incision

22. During this period in the postoperative phase, Piya Jordan should use a heating pad on her incision to promote comfort.
   a. True
   b. False

Intravenous Therapy

∞ **Reading Assignment:** Intravenous Therapy (Chapter 18)

Patient: Patricia Newman, Room 406

Objectives:

1. List the indications for intravenous fluid therapy.

2. Describe the types of fluids used for intravenous fluid therapy.

3. Describe the types of venous access devices and other equipment used for intravenous therapy.

4. Explain the causes, signs and symptoms, and nursing implications of the complications of intravenous fluid or drug therapy.

5. Explain the nursing responsibilities when a patient is receiving intravenous therapy.

Exercise 1

Writing Activity

30 minutes

1. Fluids containing water and electrolytes are referred to as _____;

   fluids containing blood and blood products are called _____.

2. Tonicity is the term used to measure the concentration of vitamins in an intravenous solution.
   a. True
   b. False

3. A nurse is preparing an adult patient for an appendectomy. Which of the following cannula sizes will be most appropriate?
   a. 14- to 16-gauge
   b. 18- to 20-gauge
   c. 22-gauge
   d. 24-gauge

4. A nurse is preparing to start an IV. Which of the following tools may be used to assist in locating a vein?
   a. Transilluminator
   b. Veni-locator
   c. Transdermal lighting
   d. Intradermal lighting

5. Indicate whether each of the following statements is true or false.

   a. _____ Presently, heparin is used to flush only central lines and not peripheral locks.

   b. _____ A round-corded tourniquet is most beneficial when starting an IV.

   c. _____ The use of normal saline injections at the IV site to provide anesthesia is a widely used practice.

6. When selecting a site for IV insertion, the nurse should begin with the most

   _____ site and move _____ as needed.

7. When preparing to start an IV, which of the following are contradictions to the use of an extremity? Select all that apply.

_____   It is the patient's dominant hand.

_____   There is impaired circulation in the extremity.

_____   There is impaired lymphatic drainage in the extremity.

_____   The patient has an AV graft in the extremity.

_____   The patient has a history of a mastectomy on the same side as the extremity.

_____   Blood work was obtained from the extremity within the last 4 hours.

8. A patient asks the nurse whether antibiotic ointment should be used at the site of her IV insertion. Which of the following is the best reply by the nurse?
   a. "There is no risk for developing an infection at the insertion site."
   b. "The cleaning of the site adequately sterilized it."
   c. "There is some controversy concerning that practice. I will need to consult with your physician."
   d. "I will apply Neosporin during my next assessment."

9. When monitoring the rate of flow for an intravenous infusion, the nurse must recognize factors that affect the infusion rate. Which of the following statements concerning intravenous infusions are correct? Select all that apply.

_____   Lowering the IV bag will increase the rate of flow.

_____   A full infusion bag will infuse more rapidly.

_____   Viscous fluids will flow more rapidly.

_____   Venting rigid containers is necessary to ensure flow.

_____   Larger cannulas will promote a more rapid rate of infusion.

10. Permission for a licensed practical nurse to administer IV push medications is determined

    by the _____ _____ _____ of the
    individual state in which the LPN is practicing.

11. Identify at least three indications for the administration of intravenous fluids.

Exercise 2

CD-ROM Activity

45 minutes

- Sign in to work at Pacific View Regional Hospital for Period of Care 2. (*Note:* If you are already in the virtual hospital from a previous exercise, click on **Leave the Floor** and then **Restart the Program** to get to the sign-in window.)
- From the Patient List, select Patricia Newman (Room 406).
- Click on **Get Report** and read the shift report.
- Click on **Go to Nurses' Station**.
- Click on **Chart** and then on **406**.
- Click on and review the **Nursing Admission** and **Laboratory Reports**.

1. Why was Patricia Newman admitted to the hospital?

2. Patricia Newman has a serum potassium level of _____ mEq/L.

3. The normal range for serum potassium levels is:
   a. 3.0-4.5 mEq/L.
   b. 3.5-5.1 mEq/L.
   c. 3.5-5.5 mEq/L.
   d. 4.0-6.5 mEq/L.

→ • Click on and review the **Physician's Notes** and **Physician's Orders**.

4. What intravenous fluids have been ordered by the physician?

5. Which of the following are roles of potassium in the body? Select all that apply.

_____   Protein synthesis

_____   Regulation of acid-base balance

_____   Maintenance of fluid osmolarity and volume within the cell

_____   Transmission of nerve impulses

_____   Metabolism of carbohydrates

_____   Synthesis and breakdown of glycogen

6. The physician has ordered the intravenous solution to infuse at _____ mL/hr.

7. Over a 24-hour period, Patricia Newman should receive _____ mL of intravenous fluids.

8. The total number of calories that will be provided to Patricia Newman from a liter of fluids is:
   a. 100.
   b. 150.
   c. 170.
   d. 190.
   e. 200.
   f. 340.

9. The intravenous solution ordered by the physician can best be described as:
   a. isotonic.
   b. hypotonic.
   c. hypertonic.

10. Based on the standards of the Intravenous Nurses Society, how frequently should Patricia Newman's IV tubing be changed? (*Hint:* See pages 288-289 in your textbook.)
    a. Every 24 hours
    b. Every 48 to 72 hours
    c. Weekly
    d. Only when problems arise

→ • Click on **Return to Nurses' Station** and then on **406**.
  • Click on **Check Armband**.
  • Review the **Initial Observations**.
  • Click **Patient Care** and then **Physical Assessment** to complete an assessment of the IV site.

11. Patricia Newman is _____ years of age.

12. Older patients may require special observations related to the administration of intravenous fluids. Identify some common issues regarding IV administration unique to the older adult population.

13. When assessing Patricia Newman's IV site, the nurse knows that which of the following manifestations are consistent with infiltration? Select all that apply.

_____ Warmth at IV site

_____ Coolness at IV site

_____ Leaking of fluid around site of cannula insertion

_____ Paleness in the skin surrounding site of insertion

_____ Edema surrounding site of insertion

14. Patricia Newman's IV site demonstrates symptoms consistent with early-onset infiltration.
    a. True
    b. False

15. If an IV site infiltrates, the extremity should be:
    a. elevated.
    b. positioned lower than the level of the heart.
    c. wrapped to prevent further absorption of fluids into the extremity's tissue.
    d. wrapped in an ice pack to prevent neurological damage.

16. Patricia Newman's IV can best be described as:
    a. peripheral.
    b. midline.
    c. PVC.
    d. PICC.
    e. CVC.

17. Review Patricia Newman's condition. What are the underlying rationales for her intravenous therapy?

→ • Click on **MAR** and review Patricia Newman's scheduled medications.

18. Identify the medication that will be administered via IV.

19. The preceding medication will be administered _____.

20. The total volume that will be infused with the IV medication will be _____ mL.

21. The IV medication is premixed in a _____ solution.

LESSON 8

Loss, Death, and End-of-Life Care

/OᴚO **Reading Assignment:** Loss, Death, and End-of-Life Care (Chapter 24)

Patient: Pablo Rodriguez, Room 405

Objectives:

1. Understand the beliefs and practices related to death and dying.

2. Describe the responses of patients and their families to terminal illness and death.

3. Identify nursing diagnoses that are appropriate for the terminally ill.

4. Identify and discuss nursing interventions for meeting the needs of terminally ill and dying patients.

5. Identify and discuss nursing interventions for meeting the needs of terminally ill patients' significant others.

6. Identify issues related to caring for the dying patient, including advance directives, do-not-resuscitate decisions, brain death, organ donation, and pronouncement of death.

Exercise 1

Writing Activity

30 minutes

1. Grief that is delayed or exaggerated may be identified as _____.

2. Match each of the following age groups with their associated beliefs and attitudes about death.

Age Group	Belief/Attitude
_____ Preschool	a. Death is seen as unavoidable.
_____ School age	b. Religious beliefs have the greatest influence on beliefs concerning death.
_____ Preadolescent	
	c. Death can be reversed.
_____ Adolescent	
	d. Fear of experiencing a prolonged death may be
_____ Young adulthood	expressed.
_____ Middle adulthood	e. Death anxiety may be experienced.
_____ Older adulthood	f. Death is the result of a violent act.
	g. Attitudes concerning death are based on those of adults in their network.

3. Studies show that sheltering children from being exposed to death and dying is an effective means of managing the situation.
   a. True
   b. False

4. After the death of a spouse, an individual may report an increase in physical disorders.
   a. True
   b. False

5. Emotional development and acceptance of a death are interrelated.
   a. True
   b. False

6. Anticipatory grief provides a healthy response to the grief process.
   a. True
   b. False

7. Arrange each Elisabeth Kubler-Ross stage of death and dying in its typical order of occurrence.

	Stage	Order of Occurrence
_____	Acceptance	a. Stage 1
_____	Bargaining	b. Stage 2
_____	Denial	c. Stage 3
_____	Depression	d. Stage 4
_____	Anger	e. Stage 5

8. While providing assistance to the spouse of a patient diagnosed with a terminal illness, the nurse notes that the individual is having difficulty making decisions and has a lack of interest in the future. Which of the following grief clusters, as defined by Martoccio, is being manifested?
   a. Shock and disbelief
   b. Yearning and protest
   c. Anguish, disorganization, and despair
   d. Identification in bereavement
   e. Reorganization and restitution

9. While working in the Emergency Department, the nurse is providing emotional support for the parents of a young car crash victim who is not expected to live. Which of the following physical manifestations and/or emotions can the nurse anticipate the parents to experience? Select all that apply.

   _____ Shortness of breath

   _____ An overwhelming sense of strength to manage the situation

   _____ Tightness in the chest

   _____ Feelings of suffocation

   _____ Feelings of emptiness

10. While working with the family of a patient who is nearing death, the nurse should use which of the following statements to facilitate the interaction? Select all that apply.

   _____ "You are being so strong."

   _____ "I know how you feel."

   _____ "I will keep you in my thoughts."

   _____ "Time will make it easier."

   _____ "You must get on with your life."

11. Which of the following may be viewed as risk factors for experiencing a maladaptive grief process? Select all that apply.

_____ Dependent relationships

_____ A lengthy terminal illness

_____ History of alcohol abuse

_____ Current history of substance abuse

_____ Cumulative grief over multiple unresolved losses

12. Written statements that identify a patient's wishes concerning medical care are known as

_____ _____.

13. What is the Patient Self-Determination Act?

Exercise 2

CD-ROM Activity

30 minutes

- Sign into work at Pacific View Regional Hospital for Period of Care 1. (*Note:* If you are already in the virtual hospital from a previous exercise, click on **Leave the Floor** and then **Restart the Program** to get to the sign-in window.)
- From the Patient List, select Pablo Rodriguez (Room 405).
- Click on **Get Report** and read the shift report.
- Click on **Go to Nurses' Station**.
- Click on **Chart** and then **405**.
- Click on and review the **History and Physical**.

1. Why has Pablo Rodriguez been admitted to the hospital?

2. What are Pablo Rodriguez's medical diagnoses?

3. Which of the following best describes Pablo Rodriguez's mental state at the time of admission?
   a. In denial
   b. Resolved to his fate
   c. Depressed
   d. Anxious
   e. Nervous
   f. Angry

- Click on and review the **Nursing Admission**.

4. Which of the following best describes the status of Pablo Rodriguez's advance directive?
   a. Pablo Rodriguez has executed an advance directive.
   b. Pablo Rodriguez has provided the hospital with a copy of the advance directive.
   c. Pablo Rodriguez has reported the existence of an advance directive and his intent to provide a copy to the hospital.
   d. Pablo Rodriguez has not executed an advance directive and does not wish further discussion regarding the matter.
   e. Pablo Rodriguez has been provided written information about his rights regarding advance directives.

5. Pablo Rodriguez is unable to provide self-consent in light of his medical and emotional condition.
   a. True
   b. False

6. In the event that a party would be required to "step forward" to assist with decision making regarding Pablo Rodriguez's medical care, who will take on this role?
   a. Pablo Rodriguez's spouse
   b. The hospital attorney
   c. Pablo Rodriguez's physician
   d. The hospital's ethics committee
   e. Pablo Rodriguez's daughter
   f. Pablo Rodriguez's son

7. In the event that religious council or sacraments are requested by Pablo Rodriguez or his family, which of the following would most likely be consulted?
   a. A protestant minister
   b. A priest
   c. A rabbi
   d. A shaman

• Click on **Return to Nurses' Station** and then on **405**.
• Review the **Initial Observations**.
• Click on **Patient Care** and then on **Nurse-Client Interactions**.
• Select and view the video titled **0730: Symptom Management**. (*Note:* Check the virtual clock to see whether enough time has elapsed. You can use the fast-forward feature to advance the time by 2-minute intervals if the video is not yet available. Then click again on **Patient Care** and **Nurse-Client Interactions** to refresh the screen.)

8. Which of the following adjectives best describes Pablo Rodriguez's ability to share his concerns?
   a. Hesitant
   b. Eager
   c. Open
   d. Nervous

9. Discuss Pablo Rodriguez's beliefs about how he became ill.

10. Pablo Rodriguez views sharing his feelings as
    a. an opportune time to bond with his loved ones.
    b. a sign of weakness.
    c. a waste of time.
    d. a key step in preparing for his death.

→ • Click on and review the **Kardex**.

11. Pablo Rodriguez has been ill for how long?

12. Pablo Rodriguez's code status is identified as
    a. full code.
    b. partial code—medications only.
    c. partial code—CPR only.
    d. DNR.

The Patient with Cancer

Reading Assignment: The Patient with Cancer (Chapter 25)

Patient: Pablo Rodriguez, Room 405

Objectives:

1. Explain the differences between benign and malignant tumors.

2. List the most common sites of cancer in men and women.

3. Describe measures to reduce the risk for cancer.

4. List nursing responsibilities for the care of patients having diagnostic tests to detect possible cancer.

5. Explain the nursing care of patients undergoing various types of cancer therapy: surgery, radiation, chemotherapy, and biotherapy.

Exercise 1

Writing Activity

45 minutes

1. Specific characteristics are used to differentiate benign cells from malignant cells. Match each of the following characteristics to the cellular category it is most closely associated with.

Characteristic	Cellular Category
_____ A distinct recognizable appearance	a. Benign
_____ Ability to perform a specific function	b. Malignant
_____ The presence of multiple nuclei	
_____ Nuclei that are large in size	
_____ Nuclei that are small in size	
_____ Cell division inhibited by inadequate space and insufficient nutrients	
_____ Cells not readily recognized by other cells	
_____ Will continue to divide despite space constraints	

2. _____ _____ is the term used to describe the movement of cancer cells into adjoining tissue.

3. List factors that may promote the transformation of normal cells into malignant cells.

4. Which of the following foods have been shown to reduce the risk for developing cancer? Select all that apply.

_____ Broccoli

_____ Lettuce

_____ Bananas

_____ Carrots

_____ Grapefruit

_____ Tomatoes

5. Indicate whether each of the following statements is true or false.

a. _____ The risk for developing lung cancer is similar among users of smokeless tobacco and cigarette smokers.

b. _____ African-American women have the highest rates of breast cancer.

6. A 21-year-old woman who is sexually active, has had negative Pap smears for the last 4 years, and has no other risk factors asks how frequently she should have a Pap smear. Based on your knowledge, which of the following time frames should the nurse give this patient?
a. Annually
b. Every 2 years
c. Every 3 years
d. Every 6 months

7. A patient asks at what age she should have her first mammogram. A review of the patient's history is devoid of any significant risk factors. What information should be provided to the patient?
a. 25 years of age
b. 30 years of age
c. 40 years of age
d. 45 years of age

8. When providing care to an African-American male, the nurse should be aware that which of the following cancers are most prevalent in this population? Select all that apply.

_____ Oral

_____ Prostate

_____ Breast

_____ Colon

_____ Integumentary

_____ Rectal

_____ Lung

9. Match each of the following diagnostic tests with its correct description. (*Hint:* Refer to pages 374-375 in your textbook.)

Diagnostic Test	**Description**
_____ Computed tomography	a. Noninvasive, high-frequency sound waves are used to examine external body structures.
_____ Radionuclide scans	
_____ Ultrasound testing	b. A computer processes radio-frequency energy waves to assess spinal lesions, as well as cardiovascular and soft tissue abnormalities.
_____ Magnetic resonance imaging	
	c. Radiographs and computed scanning are used to provide images of structures at differing angles.
	d. A substance is injected; the uptake is evaluated to identify areas of concern.

10. _____ therapy is used when a patient who has had surgery or radiotherapy is free of signs of disease but has a high risk for recurrence of the disease.

11. Prior to radiation therapy, the physician marks the skin of the patient. Which of the following instructions should be provided to the patient concerning these markings?
a. "You may wash these marks with soap and water after this treatment."
b. "Use a mild solution of rubbing alcohol and water to remove these marks."
c. "Do not remove these marks."
d. "Use lotion to soften the skin around these marks if needed."

12. A patient undergoing treatment for cancer has experienced alopecia. Which of the following should be included in information to the patient concerning this occurrence? Select all that apply.

_____ The hair color may be different after regrowth.

_____ The texture of new hair growth will mimic that of the original hair.

_____ The alopecia is temporary.

_____ Medications may assist in limiting the amount of hair lost.

_____ Alopecia may be partial or total.

13. The complete blood cell profile of a patient diagnosed with cancer shows a reduction in the number of circulating platelets. Which of the following terms is used to describe this condition?
a. Leukopenia
b. Thrombocytopenia
c. Anemia
d. Neutropenia

14. A patient undergoing radiation treatment reports that he is perspiring and asks what can be done to manage this problem. Which of the following statements should be included in information provided to the patient?
    a. "You may use deodorant but not antiperspirant."
    b. "The use of antiperspirants is allowed."
    c. "You may use corn starch to absorb the moisture."
    d. "There is nothing that can be done to manage this problem."

15. Indicate whether each of the following statements is true or false.

    a. _____   Obesity is associated with cancers of the colon, breast, prostate, and gallbladder.

    b. _____   High levels of alcohol intake are associated with cancer of the colon and breast.

16. _____ _____ is a complex metabolic problem characterized by weight loss, anemia, and abnormalities in fat, protein, and carbohydrate metabolism.

17. Nontraditional therapies combined with conventional methods are known as

    _____. Therapies used in lieu of traditional therapies are termed

    _____.

Exercise 2

 CD-ROM Activity

45 minutes

- Sign in to work at Pacific View Regional Hospital for Period of Care 2. (*Note:* If you are already in the virtual hospital from a previous exercise, click on **Leave the Floor** and then **Restart the Program** to get to the sign-in window.)
- From the Patient List, select Pablo Rodriguez (Room 405).
- Click on **Get Report** and read the shift report.
- Click on **Go to Nurses' Station** and then on **405**.
- Click on and review the **Clinical Alerts**.
- Click on **Chart** and then on **405**.
- Click on and review the **Nursing Admission** and **History and Physical**.

1. What are Pablo Rodriguez's medical diagnoses?

2. What were Pablo Rodriguez's chief complaints at the time of admission?

3. At the time of admission, what interventions were implemented to address the Pablo Rodriguez's chief complaints?

4. How does Pablo Rodriguez report his prognosis?

5. Pablo Rodriguez has a positive family history of cancer.
   a. True
   b. False

6. Based on information reported in the Nursing Admission, what physiological changes have taken place as a result of the cancer?

7. Which of the following methods of treatment does Pablo Rodriguez report using to manage his cancer? Select all that apply.

   _____ Surgery

   _____ Radiation

   _____ Chemotherapy

   _____ Alternative therapies

   _____ Complementary therapies

8. _____ is a means of cancer treatment that can be used to reduce or slow the growth of metastatic cells.

9. Which of the following best describe the modes of action and uses for radiation therapy? Select all that apply.

   _____ May be administered internally

   _____ May be administered externally

   _____ Used exclusively for palliative care

   _____ Used to treat cancer that cannot be surgically removed

   _____ Used to manage cancer that has spread to local lymph nodes

• Click on and review the **Physician's Orders** and **Physician's Notes**.

10. The physician has ordered a low-fat, bland diet. Which of the following items will Pablo Rodriguez be allowed to include in this diet? Select all that apply.

_____ Organ meats

_____ Toast

_____ Baked chicken

_____ Broth

_____ Milk shakes

_____ Tacos

11. Discuss the implications of this diet on Pablo Rodriguez's preferred foods.

• Click on and review the **Laboratory Reports**.

12. Pablo Rodriguez's hemoglobin level is reduced. Which of the following factors may be associated with the presence of anemia? Select all that apply.

_____ Dehydration

_____ A low red blood cell count

_____ A lack of hemoglobin in the erythrocytes

_____ Fluid retention

_____ Recent infection

13. Indicate whether each of the following statements is true or false.

a. _____ Pablo Rodriguez's platelet levels are abnormal.

b. _____ Pablo Rodriguez's white blood cell count is reduced, reflecting immuno-suppression.

14. Which of the following complaints voiced by Pablo Rodriguez can be attributed directly to the results reflected in the complete blood cell count?
    a. Nausea
    b. Vomiting
    c. Constipation
    d. Fatigue

15. Pablo Rodriguez had an electrolyte panel drawn. Which of his electrolyte values are abnormal? Select all that apply.

    _____ Sodium

    _____ Potassium

    _____ Chloride

    _____ Calcium

    _____ Phosphorus

    _____ Magnesium

→ • Click on **Return to Room 405**.
  • Click on **Patient Care** and then on **Physical Assessment**. Complete a head-to-toe assessment of Pablo Rodriguez.

16. At the time of his admission, Pablo Rodriguez reported being unable to tolerate oral intake. What assessment findings support this report?

→ • Click on **Chart** and then on **405**.
  • Click on and review the **Physician's Orders**.

17. What medications were ordered to manage Pablo Rodriguez's nausea?

18. The following medications have been prescribed for Pablo Rodriguez. Match each drug with its correct classification/use.

Medication	**Classification/Use**
_____ Morphine sulfate	a. Laxative
_____ Metoclopramide hydrochloride	b. Narcotic analgesic
_____ Dexamethasone	c. Schedule IV hypnotic
_____ Senna	d. Corticosteroid, systemic
_____ Lactulose	e. Laxative, ammonia detoxicant
_____ Neutra-Phos	f. Antiemetic
_____ Ondansetron hydrochloride	g. Laxative; exerts osmotic effect in small intestine
_____ Zolpidem tartrate	h. Antiemetic

19. The physician prescribed ondansetron hydrochloride for Pablo Rodriguez. Which of the following side effects associated with this medication may further complicate problems the patient is currently having? Select all that apply.

_____ Fatigue

_____ Excitability

_____ Diarrhea

_____ Urinary retention

_____ Constipation

_____ Blurred vision

20. In addition to opioids, what mediations may be used in the management of cancer pain?

Acute and Chronic Respiratory Disorders

👓 **Reading Assignment:**   Acute Respiratory Disorders (Chapter 30)
Chronic Respiratory Disorders (Chapter 31)

Patients: Jacquline Catanazaro, Room 402
Patricia Newman, Room 406

Objectives:

1. Identify data to be collected in the nursing assessment of a patient with a respiratory disorder.

2. Identify the nursing implications of age-related changes in the respiratory system.

3. Describe diagnostic tests or procedures for respiratory disorders and nursing interventions.

4. Explain nursing care of patients receiving therapeutic treatments for respiratory disorders.

5. Discuss the pathophysiology, signs and symptoms, complications, diagnostic measures, and medical treatment for acute and chronic disorders.

6. Identify examples of chronic inflammatory obstructive and restrictive pulmonary diseases.

7. Explain the relationship between cigarette smoking and chronic respiratory disorders.

Exercise 1

Writing Activity

30 minutes

1. The area in the brain that controls the respiratory system is the _____.

2. The normal respiratory rate in the adult is between _____ and _____ breaths per minute.

3. Match each of the following respiratory disorders with its appropriate description.

Respiratory Disorder	**Description**
_____ Atelectasis	a. Inflammation of the lung with consolidation and exudation
_____ Pleural effusion	b. Accumulation of fluid in the space between the visceral pleura and parietal pleura of the thorax
_____ Hemothorax	c. A collapsed or airless state of the lung or portion of a lung
_____ Pneumothorax	
_____ Pneumonia	d. An infectious, inflammatory, reportable disease that is chronic and commonly affects the lungs, although it may occur in other areas of the body
_____ Asthma	e. An inflammatory response that constricts the bronchi, causing edema and increased sputum
_____ Emphysema	
_____ Tuberculosis	f. Bleeding into the pleural space secondary to chest trauma
	g. Pathological accumulation of air in tissues or organs
	h. Air from the lung leaking into the pleural space or chest

4. During shift report, the outgoing nurse advises you that the patient is demonstrating Kussmaul's respirations. Based on your knowledge, you recognize that the patient's respiratory patterns will contain which of the following characteristics? Select all that apply.

_____ A regular pattern

_____ Periods of apnea

_____ Deep, uneven respirations

_____ A respiratory rate greater than 20 breaths per minute

_____ Tachypnea

5. After administration of an analgesic, which of the following types of respiratory patterns would you anticipate the patient to exhibit?
   a. Biot's
   b. Kussmaul's
   c. Cheyne-Stokes
   d. Tachypnea
   e. Bradypnea

6. Describe changes associated with aging that may increase the potential for complications in the elderly patient.

7. While caring for a patient demonstrating a productive cough, the nurse must record the

   characteristics of the sputum. These characteristics include _____,

   _____, _____, and _____.

8. When performing a respiratory assessment, the nurse must remember that the presence of

   flaring nostrils is a manifestation associated with _____

   _____.

9. Chest physiotherapy consists of _____, _____, and

   _____ drainage.

10. Chest physiotherapy can be performed only by a respiratory therapist.
    a. True
    b. False

11. Match each of the following respiratory sounds with its appropriate description.

Sound	Description
_____ Rhonchus	a. A high-pitched sound caused by air passing through narrowed passages
_____ Crackle	
	b. An abnormal sound similar to that made by rubbing pieces of hair between the finger
_____ Coarse crackle	
_____ Wheeze	c. A sound similar to Velcro pulling apart
_____ Pleural friction rub	d. A dry, rattling sound
	e. A grating, scratchy sound similar to a creaking shoe

12. A nurse is preparing to suction a patient. Which of the following steps/concepts should be included in the process? Select all that apply.

_____ Use clean technique.

_____ Administer oxygen before initiating the intervention.

_____ Administer oxygen after completion of the intervention.

_____ Apply suction as the catheter is withdrawn from the airway.

_____ Limit each suction attempt to 10 seconds.

_____ Complete the full cycle of suctioning before allowing the patient to rest.

_____ Document the patient's toleration of the procedure.

13. The physician has ordered percussion for a patient. For which of the following conditions would this plan be contraindicated? Select all that apply.

_____ Pulmonary embolus

_____ Asthma

_____ Pneumonia

_____ Lung cancer

_____ Bronchospasm

14. Match each of the following diagnostic tests with its correct description.

Diagnostic Test	**Description**
_____ Chest radiography	a. Radiograph of the chest taken to observe deep structures in motion
_____ Fluoroscopy	b. Removal of pleural fluid for examination
_____ Pulmonary function	c. Produces images of multiple body planes without radiation; used to detect abnormalities, lesions, and tumors
_____ Thoracentesis	
_____ Fiberoptic bronchoscopy	d. Used to screen and diagnose some respiratory disorders
_____ Magnetic resonance imaging	e. Used to visualize abnormalities, take biopsy samples of lesions, or remove foreign bodies
	f. Evaluates gas exchanges, pulmonary blood flow, and acid-base balance

15. A nurse is providing care to a patient who has had a bronchoscopy. Which of the following positions is therapeutic?
    a. High Fowler's
    b. Semi-Fowler's
    c. Supine
    d. Prone

16. A patient is demonstrating hypoventilation. Which of the following $PaCO_2$ results can be anticipated?
    a. Less than 31 mm Hg
    b. 32-40 mm Hg
    c. 40 mm Hg
    d. 47 mm Hg

17. Regarding the use of intermittent positive-pressure breathing (IPPB) treatments, which of the following statements is correct? Select all that apply.

    _____ IPPB is used to achieve maximal lung expansion.

    _____ IPPB delivers humidified gas with negative pressure.

    _____ IPPB forces air into the lungs with inhalation.

    _____ IPPB allows passive exhalation.

    _____ IPPB results in a nonproductive cough.

Exercise 2

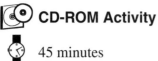 **CD-ROM Activity**

45 minutes

- Sign in to work at Pacific View Regional Hospital for Period of Care 1. (*Note:* If you are already in the virtual hospital from a previous exercise, click on **Leave the Floor** and then **Restart the Program** to get to the sign-in window.)
- From the Patient List, select Jacquline Catanazaro (Room 402).
- Click on **Get Report** and read the shift report.
- Click on **Go to Nurses' Station**.
- Click on **Chart** and then on **402**.
- Click on and review the **Nursing Admission** and **History and Physical**.

1. What are Jacquline Catanazaro's medical diagnoses?

2. Which of the following risk factors for the development of respiratory illness does Jacquline Catanazaro have? Select all that apply.

_____ Age

_____ History of travel

_____ Occupational exposures

_____ Smoking

_____ Family history

_____ Inactivity

3. Jacquline Catanazaro's racial background is typical of most asthma suffers.
   a. True
   b. False

4. When managing the care of a patient suspected of having asthma, which of the following tests may be ordered to confirm a diagnosis? Select all that apply.

_____ Complete blood count

_____ Serum electrolyte levels

_____ Arterial blood gas

_____ Pulmonary function tests

_____ Sputum cultures

→ • Click on and review the **Diagnostic Reports** and **Laboratory Reports**.

5. Jacquline Catanazaro had arterial blood gases drawn on Tuesday at 0730. Which of the following documented results were abnormal? Select all that apply.

_____ PaO_2

_____ O_2 saturation

_____ $PaCO_2$

_____ pH

→ • Click on **Return to Nurses' Station** and then on **402**.
   • Review the **Initial Observations** and **Clinical Alerts**.
   • Click on **Take Vital Signs** and review the findings.

6. What is Jacquline Catanazaro's pulse oximeter reading?

7. The pulse oximeter is a reading of the:
   a. blood's hematocrit level.
   b. oxygen saturation of hemoglobin in the blood.
   c. body's level of $PaCO_2$.
   d. body's acid-base balance.

8. When obtaining pulse oximeter readings on Jacquline Catanazaro, the nurse may use which of the following sites? Select all that apply.

_____ Ear lobe

_____ Bridge of nose

_____ Tip of the nose

_____ Finger

_____ Toe

9. A saturation reading of _____% is the critical value for oxygenation to support life.

10. Which of the following may affect pulse oximeter readings? Select all that apply.

    _____ Hypertension

    _____ Vasodilation

    _____ Hyperthermia

    _____ Dark-colored nail polish

    _____ Finger movement

→ • Click on **Patient Care** and then on **Physical Assessment** to complete a systems assessment.

11. Identify any abnormalities found during Jacquline Catanazaro's respiratory assessment.

12. If you were asked to describe the "crackles" heard in Jacquline Catanazaro's lung fields, which of the following would best describe them?
    a. Continuous sonorous sounds
    b. High-pitched musical tones
    c. Low-pitched whistling sounds
    d. Bubbling sounds

13. Another term that may be used interchangeably with "crackles" is:
    a. rales.
    b. wheezes.
    c. friction.
    d. alveolar popping.

14. The respiratory assessment reflects the presence of wheezes. Which of the following best describes the underlying cause of the wheezing sound?
    a. Pulmonary hypoventilation
    b. Mucus in the bronchioles
    c. Inflammation of the pleura
    d. Bronchoconstriction
    e. Fluid overload

15. Jacquline Catanazaro is demonstrating an increased respiratory rate. Which of the following can result in an increase in respiratory rate? Select all that apply.

_____   Exercise

_____   Fever

_____   Alkalosis

_____   Hypoxemia

_____   Hypercapnia

16. Jacquline Catanazaro's skin is noted as being moist and clammy. What significance does this have in relation to her respiratory status?

17. Jacquline Catanazaro's condition is consistent with the late phase of an asthmatic attack. Which of the following factors are present in this phase? Select all that apply.

_____   Airway inflammation is reduced.

_____   Airway inflammation is pronounced.

_____   Red blood cells have infiltrated swollen tissues.

_____   This phase typically lasts only a few hours.

_____   The patient is at a heightened risk for an acute asthmatic attack.

18. Jacquline Catanazaro is demonstrating extreme agitation. What is the impact of these behaviors on her condition?

• Click on **Patient Care** and then on **Nurse-Client Interactions**.

• Select and view the video titled **0730: Intervention—Airway**. (*Note:* Check the virtual clock to see whether enough time has elapsed. You can use the fast-forward feature to advance the time by 2-minute intervals if the video is not yet available. Then click again on **Patient Care** and **Nurse-Client Interactions** to refresh the screen.)

19. Jacquline Catanazaro is experiencing an acute asthma attack. What has been planned to manage the onset?

• Click on **Chart** and then on **402**.

• Click on the **Physician's Orders** tab and note the admission orders for Monday at 1600.

20. What medications have been ordered to manage Jacquline Catanazaro's respiratory condition? For each medication, include the dose and route of administration ordered.

• Click **Return to Room 402** and then click the **Drug** icon.

• Review the information for the drugs that have been prescribed for Jacquline Catanazaro.

21. For each medication identified in the previous question, list the mode of action.

22. When providing patient education concerning the use of beclomethasone, the nurse should tell the patient that which of the following side effects may occur?
    a. Throat irritation
    b. Productive cough
    c. Increased pulmonary secretions
    d. Skin rash
    e. Activity intolerance

23. When preparing Jacquline Catanazaro for discharge to home, which of the following concepts should be included in the education provided? Select all that apply.

    _____ Understand the prescribed drug therapy.

    _____ Limit water intake to reduce pulmonary edema.

    _____ Promptly report infections to physicians.

    _____ If symptoms occur during exercise, suspend activity.

    _____ Review potential allergens in the home environment.

Exercise 3

CD-ROM Activity

30 minutes

- Sign in to work at Pacific View Regional Hospital for Period of Care 3. (*Note:* If you are already in the virtual hospital from a previous exercise, click on **Leave the Floor** and then **Restart the Program** to get to the sign-in window.)
- From the Patient List, select Patricia Newman (Room 406).
- Click on **Get Report** and read the shift report.
- Click on **Go to Nurses' Station**.
- Click on **Chart** and then on **406**.
- Click on and review the **History and Physical** and **Physician's Notes**.

1. Why has Patricia Newman been admitted to the hospital?

2. What are Patricia Newman's medical diagnoses?

3. Potential infectious causes of pneumonia include _____,

   _____, and _____.

4. Which of the following conditions in Patricia Newman's medical history put her at an increased risk for the development of pneumonia? Select all that apply.

   _____ Smoking

   _____ Hypertension

   _____ Osteoporosis

   _____ Social isolation

   _____ Hysterectomy

   _____ Emphysema

5. Which of the following characteristics are associated with emphysema? Select all that apply.

   _____ Emphysema affects both men and women.

   _____ Symptoms typically begin to manifest while the patient is in the mid- to late 30s.

   _____ The disorder is characterized by changes in the alveolar walls and capillaries.

   _____ Disability often results in patients diagnosed with emphysema between the ages of 50 and 60 years.

   _____ Heredity may play a role in the development of emphysema.

➤ • Click on and review the **Laboratory Reports**.

6. Which of the following components of Patricia Newman's hematology test is abnormal?
   a. White blood cell count
   b. Red blood cell count
   c. Hemoglobin
   d. Hematocrit
   e. MCV
   f. Platelets

7. Assess the values from the arterial blood gases drawn on Wednesday at 0600. Which of the values are abnormal? Select all that apply.

   _____ PaO_2

   _____ O_2 saturation

   _____ $PaCO_2$

   _____ pH

8. What is the identified cause of Patricia Newman's pneumonia?

 • Click on and review the **Diagnostic Reports**.

9. The chest x-ray impression states that there are right middle and lower lobe infiltrates. Discuss how this manifestation takes place.

10. Identify several potential complications associated with pneumonia.

 • Click **Return to Nurses' Station** and then **406**.
   • Review the **Initial Observations**.
   • Click on **Take Vital Signs** and review the findings.

11. List Patricia Newman's vital signs. (*Note:* Answers will vary depending on the exact time they are taken.)

    Temperature: _____

    Heart rate: _____

    Blood pressure: _____

    Respirations: _____

➤ • Click **Patient Care** and then **Physical Assessment** to complete a systems assessment.

12. Identify findings from the systems assessment that are consistent with the diagnosis of pneumonia.

13. List several nursing interventions that could be implemented to improve Patricia Newman's airway clearance.

14. Cefotan has been ordered to treat Patricia Newman's pneumonia. Which of the following is a frequent side effect associated with this medication?
    a. Oral candidiasis
    b. Nausea
    c. Vomiting
    d. Rash
    e. Pruritis
    f. Thrombophlebitis

15. Which of the following occurrences will signal successful action by the prescribed Cefotan? Select all that apply.

_____ Increase in red blood cell count

_____ Decrease in red blood cell count

_____ Reduction in temperature

_____ Reduction in O_2 saturation

_____ Reduction in blood pressure

_____ Decrease in white blood cell count

Cardiovascular Disorders: Hypertension

/⃝⃝ **Reading Assignment:** Hypertension (Chapter 37)

Patient: Patricia Newman, Room 406

Objectives:

1. Define *hypertension*.
2. Discuss the risk factors for hypertension.
3. Identify the signs and symptoms of hypertension.
4. Understand nursing considerations of administering selected antihypertensive drugs.

Exercise 1

Writing Activity

20 minutes

1. Indicate whether each of the following statements is true or false.

   a. _____ Hypertension is more common in women than in men.

   b. _____ Hypertension occurs three times as often in African Americans as in Caucasian Americans.

2. Patients having prehypertension have systolic pressures between _____ and

   _____ and diastolic pressures between _____ and _____.

3. Identify the two factors that determine blood pressure.

4. _____ _____ _____ is the force within blood vessels that the left ventricle must overcome to eject blood from the heart.

5. Early onset hypertension may be manifested by:
   a. headaches at bedtime.
   b. early morning headaches.
   c. nasal congestion.
   d. blurred vision.

6. A prehypertensive patient is attempting to avoid hypertension. Which of the following interventions and/or lifestyle modifications will promote the patient's goal? Select all that apply.

   _____ Daily NSAID therapy

   _____ Isotonic exercise

   _____ Reduced cholesterol diet

   _____ Increased potassium intake

   _____ Relaxation therapies

7. A patient's physician is planning to use the stepped approach to control the patient's blood pressure. Which of the following statements concerning this method is correct?
   a. The patient will be placed on step 2 of therapy after diet and exercise have failed to manage the hypertension.
   b. The patient's blood pressure medications will be reduced once a therapeutic blood pressure is achieved.
   c. The four-step approach is used for only the most seriously ill patients.
   d. The step method is a means of selecting medications to treat hypertension.

8. Ethnicity can affect a patient's ability to metabolize antihypertensive medications.
   a. True
   b. False

9. What effects can antihypertensive medications have on sexual functioning?

Exercise 2

 CD-ROM Activity

40 minutes

- Sign in to work at Pacific View Regional Hospital for Period of Care 1. (*Note:* If you are already in the virtual hospital form a previous exercise, click on **Leave the Floor** and then **Restart the Program** to get to the sign-in window.)
- From the Patient List, select Patricia Newman (Room 406).
- Click on **Get Report** and read the shift report.
- Click on **Go to Nurses' Station**.
- Click on **Chart** and then on **406**.
- Click on and review the **History and Physical**.

1. Identify significant health concerns from Patricia Newman's medical history.

→ • Click on and review the **Nursing Admission**.

2. Upon admission, Patricia Newman's blood pressure was _____.

→ • Click on **Return to Nurses' Station**.
• Click on the **Drug** icon and review the entries for atenolol and chlorothiazide.

3. Patricia Newman takes atenolol 50 mg PO and chlorothiazide 500 mg PO daily to manage her hypertension. Identify the action or classification of each of these medications.

4. The normally recommended dosage of atenolol is _____ to _____ mg.

5. Patricia Newman's prescribed dosage of atenolol is within recommended limits.
   a. True
   b. False

6. Which of the following manifestations are side effects associated with atenolol? Select all that apply.

   _____ Cold extremities

   _____ Constipation

   _____ Diarrhea

   _____ Nausea

   _____ Headache

   _____ Impotence

7. Chlorothiazide is associated with excretion of which of the following electrolytes? Select all that apply.

_____ Sodium

_____ Phosphorus

_____ Potassium

_____ Zinc

_____ Calcium

_____ Magnesium

_____ Chloride

8. Discuss the interrelationship between atenolol and chlorothiazide.

9. Identify several nursing considerations for Patricia Newman in relation to the medications prescribed to manage her hypertension.

 • Click on **Return to Nurses' Station**.
• Click on **Chart** and then on **406**.
• Click on and review the **Laboratory Reports**.

10. Patricia Newman's potassium level is 3.2 mEq/L. Which of the following foods should be added to her diet to manage these levels? Select all that apply.

_____ Broccoli

_____ Lettuce

_____ Apricots

_____ Apples

_____ Blueberries

_____ Prunes

11. A normal potassium level is between _____ and _____ mEq/L.

12. The text identifies three risk groups related to hypertension. To which of these risk groups does Patricia Newman belong? (*Hint:* See page 715 in your textbook.)
    a. Group A
    b. Group B
    c. Group C

13. Patricia Newman has secondary hypertension.
    a. True
    b. False

14. Several risk factors for developing hypertension are listed below. Which of these risk factors apply to Patricia Newman? Select all that apply.

_____ Dyslipidemia

_____ Atherosclerosis

_____ Diabetes mellitus

_____ Cigarette smoking

_____ Aging

_____ Gender

_____ Obesity

_____ Sedentary lifestyle

Digestive Tract Disorders

Reading Assignment: Digestive Tract Disorders (Chapter 38)

Patient: Piya Jordan, Room 403

Objectives:

1. Identify nursing responsibilities in caring for patients undergoing diagnostic tests and procedures for digestive tract disorders.

2. List data to be included in the nursing assessment of a patient with a digestive tract disorder.

3. Describe nursing care of patients with gastrointestinal intubation and decompression, tube feedings, total parenteral nutrition, digestive tract surgery, and drug therapy for digestive tract disorders.

4. Describe the pathophysiology, signs and symptoms, complications, and medical treatment of selected digestive tract disorders.

Exercise 1

Writing Activity

30 minutes

1. The functions of the digestive tract are _____, _____,

   _____ of nutrients, and _____ of wastes.

2. Match each of the following gastrointestinal structures with its appropriate function.

Gastrointestinal Structure	Digestive Function
_____ Mouth	a. No known function
_____ Colon	b. Closes when food is swallowed to prevent aspiration
_____ Epiglottis	c. Secretes bile for the emulsification of fat
_____ Esophagus	d. Mixes food with saliva
_____ Pancreatic duct	e. Finishes digestion of chyme and absorption across a smaller number of villi, especially at the distal end
_____ Ilium	f. Reabsorbs water and electrolytes and prepares waste for excretion
_____ Appendix	
_____ Liver	g. Transports food bolus from mouth to stomach
_____ Pyloric sphincter	h. Collects pancreatic enzymes and transports them to the duodenum
	i. Prevents backflow of alkaline intestinal contents into the stomach

3. Which of the following techniques should the nurse include when examining the abdomen? Select all that apply.

   _____ The patient should be in semi-Fowler's position.

   _____ The patient should be supine.

   _____ The patient's knees should be flat.

   _____ The patient's knees should be slightly flexed.

   _____ The patient's abdomen should be thought of as divided into four quadrants.

4. When assessing for bowel sounds, the nurse should listen for at least 1 minute before recording bowel sounds as absent.
   a. True
   b. False

5. When caring for the patient who has had a gastroscopy performed, the nurse should include which of the following in the plan of care?
   a. Monitor stools for at least 2 days for the passage of white stools.
   b. Administer laxatives.
   c. Encourage fluid intake to flush the patient's system.
   d. Continue NPO until gag reflex returns.

6. A nurse is providing information for a patient scheduled to have stool specimens collected to test for the presence of occult blood. Which of the following food items may interfere with the test results? Select all that apply.

   _____ Red meat

   _____ Poultry

   _____ Milk

   _____ Orange juice

   _____ Steroids

7. When the nurse is planning food options for a patient who has difficulty swallowing, which of the following foods should be included? Select all that apply.

   _____ Lukewarm foods

   _____ Cold foods

   _____ Mildly sweetened foods

   _____ Pureed foods

   _____ Moist pasta

8. Which of the following events can increase the body's nutritional needs? Select all that apply.

   _____ Infection

   _____ Fever

   _____ Rest

   _____ Stress

   _____ Trauma

9. A patient suspected of having Crohn's disease is being educated about an upcoming fecal fat test. Which of the following should be included in the patient's preparations?
   a. A restricted fat diet for 1 week before the test
   b. Administration of a Fleet enema the day before the test
   c. NPO after midnight the night prior to the test
   d. Refrigeration of stool specimen after collection
   e. A diet of 60 grams of fat per day for 3-6 days before the test

10. To reduce the risk for aspiration after a tube feeding, the nurse should keep the head of the patient's bed elevated for how long?
    a. 15 minutes
    b. 30 minutes
    c. 1 hour
    d. 90 minutes

11. Inherited lactase deficiency is most prevalent among those in _____,

    _____, and _____ populations.

12. A patient underwent a gastric surgical procedure in which the end of the stomach was connected to the duodenum. Based on your knowledge, you recognize that the patient has had a:
    a. total gastrectomy.
    b. modified gastrectomy.
    c. Billroth I procedure.
    d. Billroth II procedure.

13. Compare and contrast gastric and duodenal ulcers.

14. Most ulcers are caused by _____ _____.

15. Match each of the following gastrointestinal disorders with its correct description.

Gastrointestinal Disorder	**Description**
_____ GERD	a. Presence of herniations in the muscular layers of the colon
_____ Candidiasis	b. An inflammatory condition of the gastro-intestinal tract causing a cobblestone-like appearance in the mucosa
_____ Gastritis	
_____ Irritable bowel syndrome	c. Episodic bowel dysfunction characterized by intestinal pain, disturbed defecation, or abdominal distention
_____ Ulcerative colitis	
_____ Crohn's disease	d. Presence of abscesses on the colon mucosa and submucosa causing drainage, sloughing, and subsequent ulcerations
_____ Diverticulosis	
	e. Backflow of stomach acid into the esophagus
	f. Fungal infection presenting as white patches on the mucous membranes
	g. Inflammation of the lining of the stomach

16. Match each of the following drugs with its use and/or action.

Drug	**Use/Action**
_____ Diphenoxylate HCl (Lomotil)	a. Interacts with acid to form a protective gel that coats ulcer surface and promotes healing
_____ Metoclopramide (Reglan)	
_____ Sulfasalazine (Azulfidine)	b. Antiinfective used to manage ulcerative colitis
_____ Nystatin (Mycostatin)	c. Decreases intestinal motility
_____ Sucralfate (Carafate)	d. Reduces secretion of gastric acid and promotes healing of ulcers
_____ Cimetidine (Tagamet)	
_____ Promethazine HCl (Phenergan)	e. Antifungal
	f. Increases the speed of gastric emptying into the small intestine
	g. Prevents and treats nausea

Exercise 2

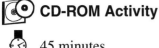 **CD-ROM Activity**

45 minutes

- Sign in to work at Pacific View Regional Hospital for Period of Care 2. (*Note:* If you are already in the virtual hospital from a previous exercise, click on **Leave the Floor** and then **Restart the Program** to get to the sign-in window.)
- From the Patient List, select Piya Jordan (Room 403).
- Click on **Get Report** and read the shift report.
- Click on **Go to Nurses' Station** and then on **403**.
- Click on **Patient Care** and then **Nurse-Client Interactions**.
- Select and view the video titled **1115: Interventions—Nausea, Blood**. (*Note:* Check the virtual clock to see whether enough time has elapsed. You can use the fast-forward feature to advance the time by 2-minute intervals if the video is not yet available. Then click again on **Patient Care** and **Nurse-Client Interactions** to refresh the screen.)

1. Based on your review of the shift report and the video, which care factors appear to be of the highest priority?

- Click on **Chart** and then on **403**.
- Click on and review the **History and Physical** and **Nursing Admission**.

2. Why did Piya Jordan initially seek care?

3. What was Piya Jordan's diagnosis after the medical examination in the Emergency Department?

4. An intestinal obstruction can be caused by a mass or by a number of other factors. List several of these factors.

5. Vomiting associated with an intestinal obstruction can lead to fluid and electrolyte imbalances and _____ _____.

6. Is Piya Jordan's intestinal obstruction considered mechanical or nonmechanical?

➔ • Click on and review the **Diagnostic Reports**.

7. Which of the following diagnostic tests were used to determine the underlying cause of Piya Jordan's condition? Select all that apply.

_____ CT of abdomen

_____ KUB

_____ Chest x-ray

_____ ECG

_____ Endoscopy

_____ Colonoscopy

➔ • Click on and review the **Surgical Reports**.

8. What were Piya Jordan's postoperative diagnoses?

9. Which of the following best describes the surgical procedure performed on Piya Jordan?
   a. Removal of the entire small intestine
   b. Removal of the entire large intestine
   c. Removal of the distal portion of the stomach and small intestine
   d. Removal of a portion of the large intestine

10. The portion of the intestine involved in Piya Jordan's obstruction was the

    _____ _____.

11. Which of the following factors put an individual at increased risk for the development of colorectal cancer? Select all that apply.

    _____ History of ulcerative colitis

    _____ History of Crohn's disease

    _____ History of hiatal hernia

    _____ High-fat diet

    _____ High-fiber diet

    _____ Family history of colorectal cancer

12. The majority of colorectal cancers are located in the rectum or lower sigmoid colon.
    a. True
    b. False

→ • Click on **Return to Room 403**.
   • Click on **Take Vital Signs**.
   • Review the **Initial Observations** and **Clinical Alerts**.
   • Click on **Patient Care** and then on **Physical Assessment**. Complete a systems assessment.

13. Piya Jordan's assessment findings reflect the greatest potential for development of postoperative complications in which of the following body systems?
    a. Respiratory
    b. Renal
    c. Integumentary
    d. Reproductive
    e. Neurological

14. Management and care of a patient who has had gastrointestinal surgery frequently includes the placement of a nasogastric (NG) tube. An NG tube has a variety of functions. Match each of the following functions with its correct description.

Function	Description
_____ Decompression	a. Irrigation of the stomach; used in cases of active bleeding, poisoning, or gastric dilation
_____ Feeding	b. Removal of secretions and gases from the GI tract
_____ Compression	c. Internal application of pressure by means of an inflated balloon to prevent internal GI hemorrhage
_____ Lavage	d. Instillation of liquid supplements into the stomach

15. Piya Jordan has had an NG tube inserted for _____.

16. Discuss responsibilities of the nurse regarding the care and management of Piya Jordan's NG tube.

→ • Click on **EPR** and then on **Login**.
• Select **403** as the patient and **Intake and Output** as the category.

17. What is the total amount of drainage from Piya Jordan's NG tube?

18. The absence of bowel sounds at this stage of Piya Jordan's recovery is normal.
   a. True
   b. False

19. When the nurse performs an assessment on Piya Jordan's abdomen, in what order should the following tools of observation occur?

Tool of Assessment	Order of Occurrence
_____ Palpation	a. First
_____ Inspection	b. Second
_____ Percussion	c. Third
_____ Auscultation	d. Fourth

Connective Tissue Disorders

Reading Assignment: Connective Tissue Disorders (Chapter 41)
Fractures (Chapter 42)

Patients: Harry George, Room 401
Clarence Hughes, Room 404

Objectives:

1. Define *connective tissue*.

2. Describe the functions of connective tissue.

3. Describe the characteristics and prevalence of connective tissue disorders.

4. Describe the diagnostic tests and procedures used for assessing connective tissue disorders.

5. Discuss the drugs used to treat connective tissue disorders.

6. Describe the pathophysiology, diagnosis, and treatment of osteoarthritis (degenerative joint disease), rheumatoid arthritis, osteoporosis, gout, progressive systemic sclerosis, and carpal tunnel syndrome.

7. Discuss the major complications, signs and symptoms, and management of fractures.

Exercise 1

Writing Activity

30 minutes

1. Rheumatoid disorders affect women more frequently than men.
   a. True
   b. False

2. _____ _____ bind structures together, providing support for individual organs and a framework for the body as a whole.

3. When performing an assessment of the musculoskeletal system, the nurse must listen for a

   crackling sound known as _____.

4. List the age-related changes of connective tissues.

5. When the patient is being prepared for a C-reactive protein test, which of the following should be included?
   a. Advise the patient to fast for 8 hours prior to the test.
   b. Obtain a clean-catch, midstream urine specimen.
   c. Restrict red meat intake the day prior to the test.
   d. Restrict fluids and food for 4 hours prior to the test.

6. When the nurse is preparing a patient for an arthrography, which of the following steps must be completed? Select all that apply.

   _____ Assess the patient for allergy to contrast agent.

   _____ Assess the patient for allergy to seafood.

   _____ Advise the patient that needle insertion may cause discomfort.

   _____ Administer a Fleet enema for patient.

   _____ Instruct the patient that swelling at the insertion site may be experienced.

7. Which of the following diagnostic tests would most likely be used to identify masses or fluid in soft tissue?
   a. Ultrasonography
   b. Tomography
   c. Nuclear scintigraphy
   d. Diskography

8. The following drugs are used in the treatment of connective tissue disorders. Match each drug with its correct classification and/or use.

Drug	**Classification/Use**
_____ Naproxen (Naprosyn)	a. Indole analogue
_____ Celecoxib (Celebrex)	b. First-generation nonsteroidal antiinflammatory
_____ Indomethacin (Indocin)	c. Second-generation nonsteroidal antiinflammatory; COX-2 inhibitor
_____ Methotrexate (Folex)	d. Used in the treatment of gout
_____ Etanercept (Enbrel)	e. Disease-modifying antirheumatic drug (DMARD)
_____ Allopurinol (Zyloprim)	f. Antiarthritic, biologic response modifiers

9. Indicate whether each of the following statements is true or false.

   a. _____ Drug therapy can provide a cure for osteoarthritis.

   b. _____ To avoid addiction, it is best that patients affected by osteoarthritis take medications only when pain is present.

10. Rheumatoid arthritis is most common in people between _____ and _____ years of age.

11. Which of the following factors are possible causes of rheumatoid arthritis? Select all that apply.

   _____ Autoimmune response

   _____ Viral links

   _____ Genetic predisposition

   _____ Reproductive history

   _____ Hormonal factors

   _____ Breastfeeding

   _____ History of osteoarthritis

12. Which of the following are clinical manifestations associated with rheumatoid arthritis? Select all that apply.

_____ Pain aggravated by movement

_____ Pain that eases within 20-30 minutes of rising in the morning

_____ Weakness

_____ Weight gain

_____ Bilateral joint changes

_____ Muscle aches and tenderness

13. Gout is a systemic disease characterized by deposits of _____

_____ in the joints and other body tissues.

14. Which of the following factors are associated with gout? Select all that apply.

_____ Genetic links

_____ Malnutrition

_____ Alcohol consumption

_____ Hypouricemia

_____ Thiazide diuretics

15. Which of the following medications may be prescribed by the physician to treat an episode of gout?
    a. Colchicine
    b. Indomethacin
    c. Corticotropin
    d. Sulfa compounds
    e. Allopurinol

16. When planning the diet of a patient with gout, the nurse should exclude which of the following foods? Select all that apply.

_____ Leafy green vegetables

_____ Gravy

_____ Sardines

_____ Organ meats

_____ Citrus fruits

17. _____ _____ _____ is a systemic disorder characterized by hardening of the skin.

Exercise 2

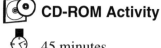 **CD-ROM Activity**

45 minutes

- Sign in to work at Pacific View Regional Hospital for Period of Care 1. (*Note:* If you are already in the virtual hospital from a previous exercise, click on **Leave the Floor** and then **Restart the Program** to get to the sign-in window.)
- From the Patient List, select Harry George (Room 401).
- Click on **Get Report** and read the shift report.
- Click on **Go to Nurses' Station**.
- Click on **Chart** and then on **401**.
- Click on and review the **Nursing Admission** and **Physician's Notes**.

1. Why has Harry George sought medical care?

2. After a medical examination, what diagnoses have been identified?

3. What factors in Harry George's medical and social history put him at risk for the development of osteomyelitis?

4. Which of the following clinical manifestations are associated with osteomyelitis? Select all that apply.

_____ Generalized pain

_____ Erythremia in surrounding tissues

_____ Wound drainage

_____ Elevated temperature

_____ Chills

➔ • Click on and review the **Laboratory Reports** and **Diagnostic Reports**.

5. Which of the following tests were ordered specifically to confirm the diagnosis of osteomyelitis? Select all that apply.

_____ Complete blood count

_____ Urinalysis

_____ Albumin levels

_____ Hemoglobin A1C

_____ Blood alcohol levels

_____ Folic acid levels

_____ Bone scan

_____ X-ray of left foot

_____ Chest x-ray

6. Which of the following laboratory values for Harry George were abnormal? Select all that apply.

_____ Red blood cell count

_____ White blood cell count

_____ Hemoglobin

_____ Hematocrit

_____ Platelets

_____ Neutrophil segs

_____ Neutrophil bands

_____ Lymphocytes

_____ Monocytes

_____ Eosinophils

_____ Basophils

7. Which of the following statements regarding Harry George's erythrocyte sedimentation rate (ESR) is correct?
   a. The ESR is decreased as a result of the infection.
   b. The ESR is increased as a result of the infection.
   c. Harry George's diabetes suppresses the ESR value.
   d. Patients with diabetes have a natural elevation in ESR.

8. Discuss the results of Harry George's x-ray and bone scan.

9. _____ _____ was identified as the pathogen responsible for Harry George's infection.

10. Harry George also has tested positive for septicemia.
    a. True
    b. False

➡ • Click on and review the **Physician's Orders**.

11. In addition to medications, what other interventions have been ordered to manage Harry George's osteomyelitis?

12. What consultations have been ordered to assist in the care of Harry George's osteomyelitis?

→ • Click on **Return to Nurses' Station** and then on **401**.

• Click on **Take Vital Signs**.

• Review the **Initial Observations** and **Clinical Alerts**.

13. Record Harry George's vital signs below. (*Note:* Findings will vary depending on exact time vital signs are taken.)

Temperature: _____

Heart rate: _____

Respiratory rate: _____

Blood pressure: _____

Pain level: _____

SpO$_2$: _____

14. Are any of Harry George's vital signs consistent with the presence of an infection? If so, which ones?

 • Click on **Patient Care** and then on **Physical Assessment**. Complete a head-to-toe assessment.

15. What findings from the assessment of Harry George's lower extremities are consistent with the diagnosis of osteomyelitis?

→ • Click on **MAR** and then on tab **401**.
  • Review the medications ordered for Harry George.

16. Which of the following medications have been ordered to manage Harry George's infection? Select all that apply. (*Hint:* Refer to the Drug Guide if needed).

_____   Gentamycin 20 mg IV

_____   Thiamine 100 mg PO/IM

_____   Cefotaxime 1 g IV

_____   Phenytoin sodium 100 mg IV

_____   Aluminum hydroxide with magnesium 15-30 mL

17. Harry George was last medicated for pain at _____. The next time that he will be able

to receive analgesics is _____.

18. Once administered, the analgesic will take effect in:
    a. 10-15 minutes.
    b. 15-30 minutes.
    c. 30 minutes.
    d. 1 hour.

19. Harry George can expect effects of the medication to last:
    a. 1-2 hours.
    b. 2-3 hours.
    c. 3-4 hours.
    d. 4-5 hours.

Exercise 3

CD-ROM Activity

45 minutes

- Sign in to work at Pacific View Regional Hospital for Period of Care 1. (*Note:* If you are already in the virtual hospital from a previous exercise, click on **Leave the Floor** and then **Restart the Program** to get to the sign-in window.)
- From the Patient List, select Clarence Hughes (Room 404).
- Click on **Get Report** and read the shift report.
- Click on **Go to Nurses' Station** and then on **404**.
- Review the **Initial Observations**.
- Click on **Chart** and then on **404**.
- Click on and review the **History and Physical**, **Nursing Admission**, and **Physician's Notes**.

1. Why has Clarence Hughes been admitted to the hospital?

2. Clarence Hughes has degenerative joint disease. This condition is also known as

_____.

3. Which of the following populations are at an increased risk for the development of osteoarthritis? Select all that apply.

_____ Small-framed patients

_____ Obese patients

_____ Older patients

_____ Individuals whose occupations require repetitive joint movements

_____ Women of childbearing age

_____ Individuals with diabetics

4. Which joints are most likely to be affected by osteoarthritis?

5. According to Clarence Hughes' admission data, he has a history of an arthroscopy. Which of the following statements concerning this procedure is most correct?
   a. The arthroscopy involves obtaining a specimen of muscle tissue for study.
   b. The arthroscopy allows the visualization of the joint cavity.
   c. After the arthroscopy there is no need to limit activity.
   d. The arthroscopy provides a definitive diagnosis for inflammatory connective tissue diseases.

6. Which of the following clinical manifestations is associated with osteoarthritis?
   a. Joint pain in the morning upon arising
   b. Bilateral joint involvement
   c. Joint enlargement
   d. Systemic involvement

7. Clarence Hughes has been taking celecoxib 100 mg PO BID to manage his osteoarthritis. Which of the following accurately describe this medication? Select all that apply.

   _____ Antiinflammatory

   _____ Used to manage allergic conditions

   _____ Inhibits platelet aggregation (clumping)

   _____ Antipyretic

   _____ Analgesic

➜ • Click on and review the **Surgical Reports**.

8. What surgical procedure was completed to manage Clarence Hughes' condition?

9. Joint replacement is avoided in patients younger than 50 years.
   a. True
   b. False

10. The life expectancy of a modern prosthesis is _____ years.

→ • Click on **Return to Room 404**.
   • Click on **Take Vital Signs**.

11. Clarence Hughes' vital signs are within normal limits.
    a. True
    b. False

→ • Review the **Initial Observations** and **Clinical Alerts**.
   • Click on **Patient Care** and then on **Physical Assessment**. Complete a systems assessment.

12. Which of Clarence Hughes' care needs are of the highest priority?

13. Which of the following interventions may be used to assist Clarence Hughes in the management of his postoperative pain? Select all that apply.

   _____ Heating pad

   _____ Massage

   _____ Relaxation techniques

   _____ Analgesics

   _____ Imagery

14. The physician has ordered the use of a continuous passive motion machine. What is the rationale for the use of this equipment? Select all that apply.

   _____ To reduce the formation of scar tissue

   _____ To promote mobility

   _____ To manage postoperative pain

   _____ To reduce the risk for infection

   _____ To lengthen the life expectancy of the prosthetic device

15. The physician has ordered Clarence Hughes to remain in bed for the first postoperative day.
    a. True
    b. False

16. During the postoperative assessment, the nurse must remain on alert for the development of complications. List several potential postoperative complications for the patient who has had joint replacement surgery.

17. Which of the following medications was ordered to manage Clarence Hughes' pain?
    a. Acetaminophen 325-650 mg PO q4-6h
    b. Temazepam 15 mg PO
    c. Oxycodone with acetaminophen 1-2 tablets PO q4-6h
    d. Enoxaparin 30 mg subQ every 12 hours

Endocrine Disorders: Diabetes Mellitus and Hypoglycemia

Reading Assignment: Diabetes Mellitus and Hypoglycemia (Chapter 46)

Patient: Harry George, Room 401

Objectives:

1. Describe the role of insulin in the body.
2. Explain the pathophysiology of diabetes mellitus and hypoglycemia.
3. Describe the signs and symptoms of diabetes mellitus and hypoglycemia.
4. Explain tests and procedures used to diagnose diabetes mellitus and hypoglycemia.
5. Discuss the treatment of diabetes mellitus and hypoglycemia.
6. Explain the differences between type 1 and type 2 diabetes mellitus.
7. Describe the complications of diabetes mellitus.

Exercise 1

Writing Activity

45 minutes

1. _____ % of the total United States population has diabetes mellitus.

2. Insulin is a hormone produced by the _____ _____ in

    the _____ of _____.

3. Normal fasting serum glucose levels are between _____ and _____ mg/L.

4. Most people with diabetes have no genetic predisposition.
    a. True
    b. False

5. Which of the following statements correctly describe the presence of insulin in the body? Select all that apply.

    _____ Insulin increases the transport of glucose into the resting muscle cell.

    _____ Insulin stimulates the conversion of glycogen to glucose.

    _____ Insulin promotes fatty acid synthesis.

    _____ Insulin inhibits the conversion of protein into glucose.

    _____ Insulin halts the storage of proteins.

6. _____ _____ _____ is diagnosed when a pregnant woman is found to have glucose intolerance for the first time.

7. Type 2 diabetes mellitus may be controlled by diet and exercise alone.
    a. True
    b. False

8. Which of the following are risk factors for the development of type 2 diabetes mellitus? Select all that apply.

    _____ Underweight

    _____ Sedentary lifestyle

    _____ Age 30 and younger

    _____ History of delivering infant weighing more than 10 pounds

    _____ African American

    _____ Latin American/Hispanic

9. The risk for diabetic nephropathy is greater for Mexican Americans than for Caucasians.
   a. True
   b. False

10. Identify at least three long-term complications associated with diabetes mellitus.

11. Which of the following should be incorporated into a foot care teaching plan for a patient with diabetes? Select all that apply.

    _____   Check feet daily.

    _____   Use heating pads instead of electric blankets for discomforts of the feet and legs.

    _____   Remove corns and calluses weekly.

    _____   Wear shoes without stockings to promote ventilation.

    _____   Wash feet daily.

    _____   Use lotion daily.

12. Diabetic ketoacidosis (DKA) is an emergency medical condition caused by an absolute

    absence of _____ .

13. When providing care to a patient with diabetes, it is necessary to assess for the use of herbal supplements that may affect blood glucose levels. Which of the following supplements may reduce the blood glucose level?
    a. Onion
    b. Dill weed
    c. Parsley
    d. Cinnamon

14. During ketoacidosis, the body breaks down _____ for energy.

15. Which of the following electrolytes is the primary concern in the management of diabetic ketoacidosis?
    a. Sodium
    b. Potassium
    c. Chloride
    d. Phosphorus
    e. Magnesium

16. Which of the following should be included in preparation for and performance of an oral glucose tolerance test? Select all that apply.

_____ The patient should consume 300-500 grams of carbohydrates for 3 days before the test.

_____ The patient must remain NPO after midnight before the test.

_____ A sweet drink is given to the patient before a blood specimen is drawn.

_____ Serving the drink cold will increase its appeal to the patient.

_____ The test can be ordered for 3- or 5-hour intervals.

17. Exercise is a successful means of reducing serum glucose levels greater than 300 mg/L.
    a. True
    b. False

18. _____ intake may be necessary during prolonged exercise.

19. Match each of the following types of insulin with its correct onset of action after administration.

Type of Insulin	Onset of Action After Administration
_____ Lantus	a. Less than 15 minutes
_____ Humalog	b. 30 minutes to 1 hour
_____ NPH	c. 1-2 hours
_____ Regular	d. 2-4 hours
_____ Ultralente	e. 4-8 hours

20. Most available insulin is U/_____.

21. Only _____ insulin can be administered intravenously.

22. Lantus cannot be mixed with other types of insulin.
    a. True
    b. False

Exercise 2

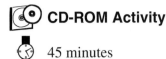 **CD-ROM Activity**

45 minutes

- Sign into work at Pacific View Regional Hospital for Period of Care 1. (*Note:* If you are already in the virtual hospital from a previous exercise, click on **Leave the Floor** and then **Restart the Program** to get to the sign-in window.)
- From the Patient List, select Harry George (Room 401).
- Click on **Get Report** and read the shift report.
- Click on **Go to Nurses' Station**.
- Click on **Chart** and then on **401**.
- Click on and review the **Emergency Department** record.

1. What is Harry George's chief complaint upon arrival to the ED?

2. When he arrived at the ED, Harry George's blood glucose level was _____.

3. Harry George has:
   a. gestational diabetes.
   b. type 1 diabetes mellitus.
   c. type 2 diabetes mellitus.

4. At 1700 the ED nurse administered 10 units of regular insulin subcutaneously. This medicine will begin to work at
   a. 1715.
   b. 1730.
   c. 1900.
   d. 1930.

5. Peak action of the insulin administered to Harry George will take place between

   _____ and _____.

6. The insulin administered to Harry George will demonstrate effectiveness until _____

   to _____.

7. The insulin administered to Harry George is considered:
   a. rapid-acting.
   b. short-acting.
   c. intermediate-acting.
   d. long-acting.

➜ • Click on and review the **Physician's Orders**.

8. The physician has ordered a(n) _____ ADA diet.

9. In this diet, what percentage of calories should come from protein?
   a. 5%-10%
   b. 10%-20%
   c. 25%-30%
   d. 30%-35%

10. Harry George should not exceed a sodium intake of:
    a. 1,500 mg/day.
    b. 2,000 mg/day.
    c. 2,500 mg/day.
    d. 3,000 mg/day.

11. What is the schedule of blood glucose checks that the physician has ordered for Harry George?

12. The physician has ordered the use of a sliding scale for Harry George's insulin coverage. Discuss the use of a sliding scale.

13. If Harry George's blood glucose is less than 150 mg/dL, his scheduled oral hypoglycemic medication will be withheld.
    a. True
    b. False

14. What impact can illness have on Harry George's diabetes?

15. Insulin dosages are based on the the total grams of _____ to be ingested.

➜ • Click on **Return to Nurses' Station** and then on **401**.
   • Click on **Take Vital Signs** and review the findings.
   • Review the **Initial Observations** and **Clinical Alerts**.

16. Harry George's fasting blood sugar at 0730 was _____.

➜ • Click on **MAR** and then on tab **401**.
   • Review the medications ordered for Harry George.

17. According to the sliding scale outlined in the Physician's Orders, Harry George should

    receive _____ units of insulin.

18. What oral medication has been ordered to manage Harry George's diabetes?

19. The medication identified in the preceding question belongs to which of the following clas-
    sifications?
    a. Sulfonylureas
    b. Meglitinides
    c. D-phenylalanines
    d. Biguanides
    e. Alpha-glucosidase inhibitors
    f. Thiazolidinediones

20. This medication works by:
    a. promoting insulin secretion by the pancreas.
    b. decreasing glucose production in the liver and increasing glucose uptake by muscle.
    c. inhibiting carbohydrate digestion and absorption.
    d. decreasing insulin resistance.

21. When administering insulin, the nurse will rotate sites. Site rotation will prevent

    _____.

Mental Health and Illness

⌒⌒⌒ **Reading Assignment:** Psychological Responses to Illness (Chapter 54)
Psychiatric Disorders (Chapter 55)

Patient: Jacquline Catanazaro, Room 402

Objectives:

1. Define *mental health*.
2. Discuss how age, cultural beliefs, and spiritual beliefs affect an individual's ability to cope with illness.
3. Identify some basic coping strategies (defense mechanisms).
4. Identify selected medications used to manage mental illness.

Exercise 1

Writing Activity

30 minutes

1. The _____ _____ includes the biologic and physio-logic aspects of a person.

2. The cognitive dimension involves the individual's ability to _____

    _____, _____ _____, and

    _____ _____.

3. List several factors that can affect an individual's ability to cope with illness.

4. After a stressful day at work, a man comes home and harshly disciplines his children. Which of the following defense mechanisms is being demonstrated?
   a. Identification
   b. Isolation
   c. Displacement
   d. Projection

5. After being sexually assaulted, the victim does not recall the events of the assault. Which of the following defense mechanisms is being demonstrated?
   a. Repression
   b. Regression
   c. Projection
   d. Denial

6. Which of the following are purposes of a therapeutic relationship (as opposed to a social relationship)? Select all that apply.

_____ It is mutually beneficial for all parties involved.

_____ It develops purposefully.

_____ Participants are not formally responsible for evaluating the interaction.

_____ The relationship has clear boundaries.

_____ The focus is on the personal and emotional needs of those involved.

7. _____ is a sustained feeling state or emotion that a person experiences in several aspects of life.

8. The external presentation of a person's feeling state and emotional responsiveness is

referred to as the _____.

9. If a patient reports seeing rats crawling on his bed, which of the following is the appropriate term for this phenomena?
   a. Illusion
   b. Dream
   c. Delusion
   d. Internal stimuli

10. A patient is seen repeatedly washing her hands. This action is referred to as an obsession.
    a. True
    b. False

11. A patient who is afraid to leave her home has a condition is known as:
    a. agoraphobia.
    b. panic disorder.
    c. obsessive-compulsive disorder.
    d. posttraumatic stress disorder.

12. A patient demonstrates a change in self-awareness. Which of the following characteristics associated with acute stress disorder is being manifested?
    a. Derealization
    b. Depersonalization
    c. Dissociative amnesia
    d. Depression

13. Indicate whether each of the following statements is true or false.

    a. _____ A somatoform disorder involves the appearance of physical symptoms with only minor physiologic dysfunction.

    b. _____ After experiencing a traumatic assault, a woman becomes unable to walk. This is an example of a panic disorder.

    c. _____ St. John's wort is commonly used to relieve depression.

14. In a _____ disorder, the symptoms are usually neurological and occur in response to some threatening or traumatic event.

Exercise 2

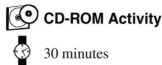 **CD-ROM Activity**

30 minutes

- Sign in to work at Pacific View Regional Hospital for Period of Care 2. (*Note:* If you are already in the virtual hospital form a previous exercise, click on **Leave the Floor** and **Restart the Program** to get to the sign-in window.)
- From the Patient List, select Jacquline Catanazaro (Room 402).
- Click on **Get Report** and read the shift report.

1. Describe the psychological behaviors documented in the change-of-shift report.

2. The anxiety being displayed can increase Jacquline Catanazaro's respiratory distress.
   a. True
   b. False

- Click on **Go to Nurses' Station**.
- Click on **Chart** and then on **402**.
- Click on and review the **Emergency Department** record.

3. According to the ED record, Jacquline Catanazaro has not been taking her prescribed

   schizophrenia medications for _____ days, and she has not been taking her asthma

   medications for _____ days.

- Click on and review the **Physician's Orders**.

4. What consultations have been ordered by the physician to assist Jacquline Catanazaro?

→ • Click on and review the **Consultations**.

5. When was Jacquline Catanazaro diagnosed with schizophrenia?

6. Schizophrenia refers to a chronic disorder in which the patient's ability to interpret the

   environment is impaired by _____.

7. Indicate whether each of the following statements is true or false.

   a. _____ The time of life in which Jacquline Catanazaro was diagnosed with
      schizophrenia is typical of the disorder.

   b. _____ After recovery from an acute exacerbation of schizophrenia, a patient may
      not return to the level of functioning experienced prior to the event.

8. What manifestations are associated with psychotic symptoms of schizophrenia?

9. Discuss the plan outlined by the psychiatrist.

→ • Click on and review the **Nursing Admission**.

10. Jacquline Catanazaro has a positive family history of mental illness.
    a. True
    b. False

11. To what does Jacquline Catanazaro attribute her lack of compliance with her prescribed medications?
    a. Financial concerns
    b. Belief that the medications are dangerous for her
    c. Concerns about the side effects of the medications on her weight
    d. Inability to remember to take medications

12. Where does the majority of Jacquline Catanazaro's social support come from?
    a. Her ex-husbands
    b. Her sister
    c. Her adult children
    d. Her parents

13. Discuss Jacquline Catanazaro's use of alcohol and/or drugs.

14. How has the exacerbation of the patient's illness affected her sleep patterns?

15. Evaluate Jacquline Catanazaro's participation in her care at the time of her illness.
    a. Active participant
    b. Moderately active participant
    c. Passive in participation with her care

16. What are Jacquline Catanazaro's primary concerns about being admitted to the hospital?
    a. Fear of losing independence
    b. Financial responsibility for hospital bills
    c. Fear of being poisoned by the medications prescribed
    d. Inability to be discharged in a timely manner

→ • Click on **Return to Nurses' Station**.
   • Click on **MAR** and then on tab **402**.

17. _____ has been prescribed to manage Jacquline Catanazaro's schizo-phrenia.